You Are Not Broken

A Compassionate Guide to
Uncovering Inner Wisdom and Transforming
Your Life with Hypnotherapy

Sara Raymond

Hypnotherapist and Somatic Life Coach

with contributing author Leah RS Braun

©2024 by Sara Raymond

All rights reserved. No part of this publication may be reproduced or transmitted in any form or by any means, electronic or mechanical, including photocopying, recording, or any other information storage and retrieval system, without the written permission of the author or publisher.

Internet addresses given in this book were accurate at the time it went to press.

This book is intended as a reference volume only, not as a medical manual. The information given here is designed to inspire and inform. It is not intended as a substitute for any treatment that may have been prescribed by your doctor. If you suspect that you have a medical problem, we urge you to seek competent medical help.

Printed in the United States of America

Published in Hellertown, Pennsylvania

Cover and design by Anna Magruder

Library of Congress Control Number available upon request

ISBN: 979-8-89420-027-9

Table of Contents

Introduction 5

Chapter 1: I Wasn't Broken, But I Sure FELT That Way 20

Chapter 2: Getting into the Right State of Mind: How Hypnotherapy Works 34

Chapter 3: Getting Started with Hypnotherapy. 53

Chapter 4: Principles of the Mind 63

Chapter 5: Your Past Doesn't Have to Determine Your Future . 76

Chapter 6: Introduction to Parts Work and Internal Family Systems in Hypnotherapy 89

Chapter 7: Who Are Your Protectors Guarding? (Hint: Your Inner Child) 98

Chapter 8: Connect with Your Inner Child 114

Chapter 9: Forgiveness and Re-Parenting Your Inner Child. . 124

Chapter 10: Preparing for Change 134

Chapter 11: Letting Go of Old Patterns, Emotions, and Behaviors 142

Chapter 12: New Roles for Your Old Parts 150

Chapter 13: Getting the Life You Want 158

Chapter 14: So What Now? (Hint: Support, Integration, Consistency) 167

Introduction

Nurturing Your Mind Like a Garden

Imagine you have a patch of grass in your backyard that you'd like to turn into a productive vegetable garden. You wouldn't judge it or be upset with it for being grass instead of a vegetable garden. The grass is there because it was planted and has served a purpose, perhaps preventing soil erosion or providing a soft place to walk.

In the process of transforming this patch of grass into a thriving vegetable garden, you wouldn't get frustrated with the grass for being there; instead, you would approach the process with patience and understanding. You would recognize the value it once provided and gently begin the process of change.

To start, you would carefully remove the grass, pulling it out by the roots to ensure it wouldn't grow back. This process might take time and repeated effort, but by doing it mindfully, you would create space for new growth. Once the soil is clear, you would plant new seeds, nourish them, and watch them flourish. You might have to go back and continue to pull out any grass sprouting up.

Similarly, the behaviors and habits you have today were adopted to protect you, keep you safe, or meet your needs at different times in your life. They grew strong because they were frequently reinforced. The same approach used for transforming the grass into a vegetable garden can be applied to your mind. By compassionately removing unhelpful thoughts and behaviors, you make room for positive, nurturing beliefs to take root.

In this book, I will guide you through a process akin to transforming a patch of grass into a beautiful garden. You will learn to recognize and gently uproot the mental "weeds"—those negative thoughts and maladaptive behaviors that no longer serve you. You will then plant and nurture new seeds, cultivating positive qualities and behaviors that align with the life you want to live.

Just as a garden requires regular care and attention, so does your mind. Through mindfulness practices, meditation, and hypnotherapy, you can tend to your mental garden, ensuring it remains vibrant and healthy. This book offers a compassionate framework for making these changes, helping you to uncover the wisdom and answers that already lie within you.

As you take this journey, remember that the process of change is ongoing. There will always be new weeds to clear and new seeds to plant. By approaching this work with kindness and patience, you can cultivate a life filled with beauty, balance, and fulfillment.

In today's stressful world, the importance of caring for our minds cannot be overstated. Just as we exercise and eat nutritious food to maintain our physical health, we must provide our minds consistent and thoughtful care to maintain our mental health.

As Thich Nhat Hanh once said, "The seeds that are watered frequently are those that will grow strong."

You Are Right Where You Need to Be

Come, sit with me—all parts of you are welcome. I invite you to make yourself comfortable. Feel safe, feel at home. If we were meeting for a personalized session, I'd meet you where you are emotionally, and together we would move at a pace that allows you to build trust: trust in me, trust in yourself, and trust in the process.

You can bring the Perfectionist within you. You can show up with your relentless Overachiever. If you have an Inner Judge or harsh inner critic, they are welcome here too. Everything about your work, family, and hobbies tells me how very *much* you've accomplished. Well done. Welcome, Anxious One. I can almost feel the continual knots in your stomach, and it's okay for now. All parts of you are welcome right here, right now with acceptance and compassion.

Maybe after all the striving and appearances, what you *really* feel is tired, exhausted even. You may also feel resentful or turned inside out trying to be what everyone else needs you to be. You cannot or do not connect with who you are or what you want. You might also feel chronically time starved and money starved, and so frazzled that you are on the verge of burnout!

If you "armor up" with achievements and perfectionism, feel like you're never good enough, or believe that it's crucial to *look successful on the outside at all times*, this book is definitely for you. Being relaxed, open, and exploratory might be the hardest thing you ever do in hypnotherapy. If you feel safe enough, let down your guard for this process.

Some of my clients have very tender and traumatic stories that might explain where they are in their current struggles. Other clients come from picture-book families that appeared healthy and caring on the outside—but the parents couldn't meet the child's emotional and other needs. No matter how you got to this place of turmoil in your life, it's okay to want and ask for help with creating something different.

I wrote this book for *you* so that you have a detailed snapshot of how hypnotherapy can help you release many of the things that are causing your overwhelm and fatigue. I will also help you release guilt, shame, trauma symptoms, anxiety, self-doubt, or fear-related silence. Hypnotherapy can guide you to discover *why* you feel overwhelmed, plus help you unwind your emotions and circumstances so that they feel manageable. With hypnotherapy, you can learn to navigate *all* of your human feelings rather than trying to escape them with more "doing."

If you desperately want to feel more ease, less pressure, and the freedom to finally be yourself (whoever the heck that is), then this book is deeply, profoundly for *you*, you beautiful, burned-out Perfectionist. I can show you how to *stop the relentless "doing"* and finally believe you are enough as you are.

The most rewarding part of my job is to help my clients—even the ones who feel helpless to make a change—to look clearly, soulfully, and tenderly at themselves. They discover their long-buried and unvalidated emotions, plus the life events and inner beliefs that hold them back from achieving their goals. Their stories are incredibly inspirational and relatable, and I'm excited to share them with you.

Note: The client stories I use in this book are an amalgamation of both true and hypothetical details and circumstances. You'll see a general snapshot of the type of people I work with who benefit most from my help. (Of course, names have been changed to protect their identity and anonymity.)

Guiding Lights of Transformation

Just like my clients, you are capable of change. Much like an acorn has everything inside its tiny little shell to become a strong and tall oak tree, *you* have within you all the resources you need to evolve, grow, and change. But in order for the acorn to become an oak tree, it must meet some resistance and pressure to finally crack open and reach for the sunlight. In the same way, your most challenging struggles are opportunities for your most profound growth. The acorn needs sun and nourishment from outside itself. In your case, sometimes it takes one or several supporting hands before you're able to see what's inside you and figure out how to put those gifts to real use in your life.

As a guide, I'm one of those supporting hands. I help my clients approach transformation from a perspective where they realize they're already *whole and enough*, rather than assuming they're broken and unredeemable.

Another simple yet important point that will be woven throughout this entire book is that *all humans are self-correcting, and you are no different.* The Hakomi Somatic Method articulates this well in Core Principles of Organicity. According to the Hakomi Institute, *"The organicity principle assumes that when all the parts communicate within the whole, we naturally self-direct, self-correct, and self-actualize."*

Our mind's job is to move us toward feeling good, safe, healthy, and vibrant. Hypnotherapy frees your mind to do what it is *designed* to do from birth, no matter your background, upbringing, culture, or parentage.

We are not in my office together, but my intention for you and this book is exactly the same as it would be for a personalized session. I invite you to adopt this self-correction, self-directing intention as you continue reading. You are an expert in you and you have the answers you seek.

Many people hear the word "hypnotherapy" and think about large auditoriums in Vegas filled to capacity with entertainment seekers sitting in front of a performer in a sequined dinner jacket.

Let's stop that image right there in its tracks. While stage and entertainment hypnotists can provide an engaging evening of fun, hypnotherapy is a wholly different (and scientifically proven) therapeutic modality. It helps thousands of struggling clients find peace, calm, confidence, and transformative behavior change every day.

As you'll discover, you're always in charge of how this process plays out for you. With every client I see, I make sure to clarify that they have a choice about the pacing and depth of the process; that's how trust and confidence start to develop between us and with yourself. You decide what's most important to you during our time together. You decide how deeply we explore those issues as I help you sink into your most relaxed and open state of mind. For healing, a slow pace is imperative so that the healing can be integrated and embodied over time. The journey of this book is no different; take it slowly and at a pace that feels safe enough for you.

Hypnotherapy is gentle. It's also effective and efficient, which are attractive qualities to my high-achieving clients. Old habits and mindsets die hard. They have become habits because they once worked well enough to keep you safe and feeling loved. But now you're ready for something different. The old ways just don't work as they once did. In fact, your outmoded mindsets and coping skills are *hurting you more than they help you now*.

Hypnotherapy Works—Trust the Process

I trust in the process of hypnotherapy because I've experienced it from both sides—as the client, and as the therapist. My own profound transformation with this modality is what guided me to help others in this way.

I came to this powerful method as a worn-out, hyperachieving mom, wife, and business owner. I had all the right success markers but could not feel any sense of contentment with all I had accomplished. I wanted to experience *real* satisfaction in my life, and I had no idea how to begin. I didn't have a particularly traumatic past, yet there were hypervigilant and overworking parts of myself keeping me exhausted and unfulfilled.

Hypnotherapy was the tool that supported me out of relentless ladder climbing and keeping up with the Joneses. I found, through hypnotherapy, that I wasn't broken, just misdirected. It took the gentle process of hypnosis to recalibrate my inner compass, listen to my deeper knowing, and *trust myself* to rewrite my inner messaging. Finally, I could transform my thoughts and behaviors little by little until I had a life I loved.

I am and will continue to be a work in progress, and I sometimes still find myself striving for an impossible state of perfection. I find myself continuing to come back to this process of hypnotherapy when I need it, because *hypnotherapy works—the magic is waiting for you.*

My clients' lives change for the better because of the profound support I offer with hypnotherapy along with the work they are willing to put in for themselves. Together, we can facilitate groundbreaking discoveries, forge subtle yet powerful connections between ideas, and improve your behaviors, personal beliefs, and attitudes.

If you have ever wanted to change your life—if you have ever been curious about hypnotherapy as a way to start—then this book is for you. I'll walk you through how to get the most out of hypnotherapy step-by-step, in a way that is self-paced. Self-hypnosis like this is how I began my journey. When I was ready, I sought deeper layers of in-person guidance from a practitioner I trusted.

When you read on, you'll come to understand the hypnotherapy process, what to expect, and whether it could be part of a healing and transformative mosaic of resources in your life. I know you want *more* out of this life, but your constant striving and *doing* doesn't offer anything in the way of peace, calm, or contentment, let alone joy. I have been there myself. This book is a wonderful gateway to a complete healing process. You'll feel more confident about whether or when to begin a therapeutic collaboration.

Here's How to Tell If This Book Is for You

- You've been feeling anxious, depressed, or scared, and want to understand and mitigate those feelings.

- You have a trauma story from your past you know is affecting your current behaviors and experience.

- You have a seemingly "normal" upbringing with few traumatic events, and can't understand why you feel so frequently burned out.

- You struggle with loving or accepting yourself as you are.

- You don't know how to silence the critical or punishing voices in your head.

- You notice that self-doubt has crept into more decisions than you would like.

- You experience a state of overwhelm from situations that used to feel manageable.

- You have a lot to be proud of in your life, but your self-criticism keeps getting louder, not quieter.

- You know that keeping up with trends and appearances is exhausting and expensive—but you can't stop chasing the next shiny thing in the hopes it will finally lead to satisfaction.

- You often feel like an imposter in your own life. You can't be who you are in relationships or your career, even though you desperately want to.

- You've become so used to living up to other people's expectations that it's hard to know what *you* want.

- You notice an anxious stomach, tense shoulders, headaches, low back pain or hip pain, or shallow breathing, or you feel like you're frequently "leaving" your body or numbing out your feelings.

- You struggle with behaviors and habits you know aren't healthy—but cannot stop them no matter what you try.

- You wonder why you always attract the "wrong" relationships with needy people who turn you inside out with their demands that you cannot seem to refuse.

This book is also for you if you have "symptoms," like imposter syndrome, lack of confidence, harsh inner judgment, perfectionism, extensive striving, or procrastination. These "symptoms" are all more accurately thought of as *safety strategies*, patterns of behavior that we adopt designed to keep us safe and comfortable, to even out our emotions, and to help us fit in—because humans need to feel a sense of belonging in order to survive.

For most people, these safety strategies do their job really well, until they don't anymore. We develop these behaviors and strategies as children, and we keep them because they *work* for a while, maybe even a long while. So if you identify as a Perfectionist, Procrastinator, or People Pleaser, or you feel like an imposter in your own life, it's likely that your safety strategies have outlasted their use.

SAFETY STRATEGIES IN ACTION

Jessica is struggling with perfectionism, which leads to a lot of inner judgment and then procrastination. She grew up in a household where both of her parents worked a lot. She often was expected to care for her younger sister. Jessica's mom was emotionally unavailable and had extremely high standards for Jessica's academic achievements. Her dad was a functioning alcoholic who could explode in anger at any moment. Jessica learned from a very young age that there was no room for her to make a mistake for fear of her mom's rejection and her dad's anger. She adopted the safety strategy of needing to be perfect to meet her needs for safety, love, and belonging in her family of origin.

Jessica could tell by the way her father opened a door whether an explosion was coming. She developed such a keen awareness, perhaps even a hyperawareness, for the emotional temperature in her home that she could respond before most people would even know something was wrong. Jessica could control, caretake, or otherwise manipulate the conditions, and be "perfect" in appearance, achievements, perception, and anticipation so that she could feel a greater sense of safety and control in her home around her family.

In her adult life, these safety strategies actually hold her back rather than keeping her safe. Now her keen hyperawareness keeps her in self-doubt around her colleagues at work. This coping skill makes her second-guess every decision. She doesn't trust anyone else to do the same quality of work she produces, so her plate is always overflowing since she will never delegate anything to her team.

At home, she anticipates doom often and rushes in to cater to her husband's emotions while micromanaging her children. She never lets them feel a sense of their own independence. She is uncertain about how to handle other people's emotions, so she tries very hard not to be the reason for any big emotions.

If you can relate to Jessica even a little bit, it's time for a new approach to getting what you really want in your life. Maybe you're not even sure yet what you want. That's okay. By the time we finish the journey of this book together, you'll realize you get to want what you want, not what everyone else thinks is the best for you.

YOUR TURN: HOW TO USE THIS BOOK

In Chapter 1: You'll learn more about me and how I found hypnotherapy. Be sure to look for themes and threads in my story that relate to *your experience*. Part of the value of others' personal stories is that we can often find something of relevance for ourselves in them. Notice if you relate to the types of struggles I've navigated as an Overachiever and Perfectionist and the ways those behaviors served as safety strategies for me for so many years.

In Chapter 2: We'll cover how hypnotherapy works so that you can clearly discern what is myth and what is truth about hypnosis. We'll also cover four different brain states and how each one works in your life. Plus you'll learn about the safety and efficacy of hypnosis and how you are always in charge of the experience, even when you allow yourself to sink into a suggestable state of mind. (Note: It's paramount that all my clients feel safe and comfortable with the hypnosis experience before we begin. Knowledge is power and builds trust over time.)

In Chapter 3: I'll lead you through my extensive intake process so that you can begin discovering and targeting the core beliefs that you may wish to change through the hypnotherapy process.

In Chapter 4: You'll learn the Principles of the Mind and how to use them to deepen your understanding of transformation. You'll connect more dots in your own experience and use these key principles to get familiar with your core beliefs and perhaps even start changing some behaviors you find problematic.

In Chapter 5: We'll walk through the developmental emotional milestones that make up our fulfillment (or lack thereof) and uncover what may be missing for you. (Don't worry—*every* human has a missing milestone or two.) The good news is that we can give these milestones to ourselves as adults, even if we missed out on them as children!

In Chapter 6: I'll show you how the ideas offered by Internal Family Systems and other Parts Work methods and hypnotherapy go hand in hand as you take a look at the different "parts" of you. You'll understand what your Protector Parts are and how they function to keep you feeling safe and loved. These parts are the ones that have set up your safety strategies from early childhood into adulthood. You'll also learn how to spot a part whose job needs to change because the way it's been "helping" you in life isn't making you feel good anymore.

In Chapters 7, 8, and 9: You'll learn who your Protector Parts are guarding: your inner child. You'll understand and practice how to identify, connect with, and re-parent your inner child. These chapters are the real substance of the hypnotherapeutic process and will enable you to finally make the sustainable mindset and behavior transformations you seek.

In Chapter 10: Now that you've identified and connected with your inner child, the way becomes clear to change your inner beliefs. You'll identify the precise beliefs that have held you where you are. You'll create new and more accurate beliefs about who you are and how you want to live.

In Chapter 11: You'll put those new beliefs in action by first letting go of the old ones. We'll do this together through journaling and ceremony. And you can continue to practice releasing old beliefs and integrating new ones by staying self-observant and taking gentle action each day to retire your "old" safety strategies. I'll show you how.

In Chapter 12: You'll learn how to reassign your Protector Parts to "new" roles within you, ones that help you achieve what you truly want in your life. You'll practice doing this with full trust in yourself to implement the changes you seek for yourself.

In Chapter 13: You'll create a deep, meaningful, and, most of all, *attainable* vision for the life you want to live. This could mean rewiring your relationships, reaching for a better job or different career, inviting adventure into your life, or even becoming the parent you've always wanted to be to your children.

Throughout the whole book: Read each chapter slowly, taking time throughout the book to move through the activities, journal prompts, and hypnosis processes I'll provide for you. Talk to your safe friends and loved ones about what you discover.

Each chapter will contain many tools to help you work through this process on your own, including:

- An "in Action" section sharing relevant and relatable stories
- A "Your Turn" section offering activities, hypnosis practices, and exercises to help you apply what you are learning
- A "Go Deeper" section with reflection questions and affirmations

When you practice the hypnosis skills I teach in this book that will guide you to go within, you will learn how and when to:

- *Trust* the messages, solutions, and guidance you find within yourself.
- Listen to any resistance that shows up, such as distraction, avoidance, or a relentless wandering mind—which is often your brain employing more outmoded safety strategies.
- Request the right sort of help at the right time outside of yourself to gain maximal relief, clarity, and empowerment so that you can finally live the life you most want.

I'm so glad you're here, and I acknowledge the bravery you're showing in your willingness to try something new. Getting vulnerable enough to look within to see what's below the surface can feel daunting, to say the least, but it's worth it.

Let's explore together how hypnotherapy can help you heal the wounded self within and consistently bring your inner "adult" to bear in all of your present challenges. This can help you feel more confident, less afraid of conflict, and more secure in speaking up for what you want out of life (and getting it).

Chapter 1

I Wasn't Broken, But I Sure FELT That Way

My hypnotherapy journey was about getting to know myself, my True Self. So many of our failures come from self-doubt. Most babies are born believing they are worthy of care and love, but certain events can take that belief away. Self-belief is fragile, and it takes only a couple of missteps to erase all of our early successes in our minds.

For me, I had lived a life of competence and achievement, but none of those accomplishments resulted in the feeling of worthiness and belonging I was seeking. Throughout my childhood, I had internalized the belief that *I wasn't worthy of love unless I was achieving*. But all the achievement was wearing me out!

Achievement was my main safety strategy—and by the time I hit age thirty-five, that safety strategy stopped working so well. I had a great family, a thriving business, a storied academic record, and many of the bells and whistles a middle-class lifestyle affords. But I felt exhausted, overwhelmed most of the time, and unclear about what I wanted in life! I often wondered, "Why has what's worked to make me feel enough for so long now make me feel so terrible all the time?"

I desperately needed a reminder that I was enough. I needed someone to show me that I wasn't broken and I had everything I needed inside myself. I needed to know I was worthy to feel loved, to be understood, and to be accepted. There was nothing I had to achieve externally to have this innately human status. My worth (and yours) is inherent and can never be taken away.

In fact, I was not broken or defective during that super-hard time in my life—just a little misguided. Remember, as we journey through this process together that you are not broken, and you do not need to be fixed, no matter how bad it appears. Before I got to this place of understanding, though, I had to run my own gauntlet of self-doubt, discontent, and low-grade, relentless "awful." My life appeared so . . . together. Why couldn't I feel as happy as I pretended to be?

Imposter syndrome was running my life. We hear about it all the time on podcasts and in blogs or magazines, but what does it mean to feel like an imposter? At first glance, imposter syndrome can feel like a general lack of confidence, like when you get up in front of people to teach a skill or talk about an area of expertise and then you doubt you have anything useful or meaningful to share.

It's normal to feel a lack of confidence in your first year of doing anything. But when you still feel that way after ten years of experience, skill building, and education, that's no longer just your confidence flagging. It's a deeper sense of being a fake or a phony, even when your expertise can back up what you say and do.

I turned thirty-five in 2015. Like many others from the picturesque planned community of Columbia, Maryland, where I grew up, I checked all the boxes. College education? Check. Great marriage and two healthy kids? Check, check. I even celebrated ten years as a successful business owner, running a thriving Pilates studio. I felt healthy and satisfied—sort of. There were no extreme feelings in my life, positive or negative. No lows, but also no highs. I met all the "shoulds" in my life with resignation, and climbed all the ladders our culture presents as signs of adulthood.

But all those "shoulds" started catching up with me. I felt caught in a cycle of relentless searching, but never finding. I thought that contentment was just around the corner—in the next yoga or Pilates training, in the next big furniture or car purchase, or the next life upgrade. I compared myself to others with heartbreaking frequency and always came up short. No "next thing" ever made me happy.

I chased and chased, but never caught up with the satisfaction I sought. The chase only made me hungrier and more exhausted. You might call it the "I'll be happy when . . ." cycle—I kept looking for happiness and contentment from things outside myself when really, all the answers were inside me.

Overachieving was a safety strategy for me. The perpetual busyness I sought allowed me to bypass the painful emotions inside me (like fear, loneliness, and despair) so I could attempt to be "good enough." I didn't know it at the time, but this strategy was a biologically appropriate pattern I developed as a child to get the love, attention, and recognition I so deeply desired but didn't receive in the way I truly needed. I am clear that my parents loved and cared for me the best way they knew how, but still I didn't feel seen and understood much of the time.

It will be crucial for you as you read this book to look back into your own safety strategies with curiosity. Overachieving became my go-to coping skill in my childhood home. Here's a brief explanation of why this happened for me:

My mom had insecurities about herself, as most people do, and sought feelings of enoughness through a high-powered job in corporate finance. Her insecurities also surfaced frequently in our daily lives as the need for her children to keep the house clean and organized, earn excellent grades, and perform well in sports. I internalized these high expectations as criticisms of me. (We'll get into how this happens and how we internalize and create inner beliefs from the care or lack thereof we received as kids.) On top of that, my dad suffered from feelings of inferiority, as in never feeling quite good enough. This showed up as seeing problems where no problems existed. For example, I would come home after winning a volleyball game and he would suggest it might be time to add in some weight training so we could continue to win games. Again, I internalized his inner messaging as a reflection on *me*—like something was wrong with me; I was the problem and I needed to be fixed.

As we move forward through the hypnotherapeutic process, you may notice many of your safety strategies coming to light. It's essential to remember that there is nothing wrong with you. These safety strategies we *all* use have a purpose: to keep us safe and secure. It's likely that you've already begun to realize that your coping skills have overstayed their welcome and no longer help you feel safe. They make you feel terrible instead, which means you're reading precisely the right book at the right time! Remember to offer yourself compassion for these safety strategies because they were adopted at a young age when you didn't have the resources and understanding you have now as an adult.

When we rejoin thirty-five-year-old-Me, I had spent seventeen years making important, life-altering decisions about marriage, family, and work following the "shoulds" in my head—and those opinions were not even mine! I didn't even know what my voice sounded and felt like, and I had to find out.

Up until this point in my life, I believed that all of my happiness and fulfillment must come from somewhere outside of myself. This belief wasn't working, as evidenced by my frustration, low mood, and confusion.

To really begin to change, I had to begin telling myself that I had everything I needed within me to find happiness and satisfaction. The external trappings didn't change what's true inside. I was enough!

And then I had to ask, Do I even want to be here? ("here" being the "right" house, in the "right" family, with the "right" kids, doing all the "right" things). Well, yes. I loved my life. I honestly wouldn't change anything significant. I needed to change the approach I was bringing to my actions, and where I was coming from. I needed to change the driving motivation and beliefs in order to release the constant striving and frantic approach to trying to be good enough.

I woke up to realize that what I really wanted was to have some say, some influence, some choice in the direction I was going! I wanted to feel it all, the highs and lows, even the painful emotions. Even though this is what I desperately wanted, I didn't know how to release the protective strategies, be more vulnerable, and allow myself to feel all the feelings safely.

This is the "good enough" that so many people—perhaps women especially—struggle with every single year. We get the stuff we're supposed to want, but the gratitude and fulfillment don't follow. The knowing that we are good enough, just as we are, is missing. Then we wake up feeling empty, forever searching for the thing that will finally land us in joy, fulfillment, impact, confidence, power, belonging, connection, or influence.

The Way Forward

The way forward is a deep and fearless dive into you, not what's outside of you. The way forward is understanding what drives you as a unique, expressive, loving, passionate human being, including all of your parts.

So let the pressure you feel today move you in a different way. When you're about to collapse under the next deadline at work or when your perfectionism gets on every last nerve of the people who love you, it's an invitation to explore. It's those moments that are inviting you inward, and it's time to listen.

Hypnotherapy is a very powerful way to begin listening. You'll discover who you are at your core and what you can do when you operate not from your head, but your heart. This process allows us to go deep below the surface of what our conscious, logical mind knows.

Our minds are more powerful than we may ever fully understand. Hypnotherapy helps us dive into the mystery and actually come out with some answers. Maybe right now you're thinking, "Yeah, right. Sure, I have everything I need inside me. Then why isn't my life perfect right now? Why aren't I calmer and finally content? Why do I look like I have it all but feel completely empty inside? Is all that inner power only available to people who closet themselves inside meditation caves and eschew polite, conventional society? Who don't have jobs or families or obligations? C'mon!"

You can absolutely harness your inner power without giving up your day-to-day life. The trick is to uncover your power and agency in a way you can actually believe. Lasting transformation happens in tiny steps that feel . . . real. Continue reading to see how it works and try it for yourself.

Lasting Change in Action

Here's an example of how change can be short-lived even with the best of intentions. You can spend all day saying to yourself, "Okay, I believe I can have a million dollars" (if that's what you truly want). So why isn't it showing up in a big bucket of bills?

It's not enough just to say that you believe you can have the thing you really want. You must first discover the conflicting belief that is holding you back from what you want. You'll then need to spend days practicing that new mindset, connecting with and cultivating the feeling of having what you want, taking consistent action to get closer to your goal, and enlisting the support you need to get there gently and joyfully, not resignedly. You don't have to do it alone, and none of us should, either.

I have committed my life's work to helping people understand their minds through hypnosis, meditation, and transformative life coaching. Through these practices, my clients can finally experience their miraculous gifts (we all have unique ones), fully use their genius (it's in there, I promise), and open the door to all the pleasure, fulfillment, confidence, and contentment available to them (which is a *lot*).

Looking Within Myself

Ironically, by the time I "discovered" meditation for myself, I had been teaching yoga and Pilates for almost ten years as a self-proclaimed nonspiritual, "all about the exercise" type of teacher. In fact, yoga is primarily an inner practice. It can be good exercise, of course, but the best yoga practice will place a huge emphasis on meditation and mindful movement.

I learned about all of that in my teacher training, but never practiced it myself. (Who had time? Being still and contemplative is hard.) I also never taught meditation to my students, because I found the prospect awkward and uncomfortable. I would focus solely on the exercise and leave the philosophy, the lessons, the present moment, and the meditation behind. Savasana, a period of relaxation, breathing, and stillness at the close of each class, was the most difficult part for me.

By the time I turned thirty-five, I was not only noticing my inability to make the changes I desired in my mindset and state of being; I also began seeing my students and fellow instructors struggling with similar issues. The universe has a way of continuously putting the same lesson in front of you, featuring a different cast of characters each time, until you finally learn the lesson and make a shift. When you find yourself saying, "Why does this keep happening to me?" it's time to pause and take note.

So I began doing the scary thing and embracing all of my yoga teachings. I had to walk the walk myself before I could help others learn the relaxation and peace that yoga promises.

You cannot separate your mind from your body for very long without feeling depleted, bereft, depressed, anxious, hopeless, and blah. And when you do finally start integrating your head and your heart, it can definitely be challenging as you begin to see and feel the things you were hiding from. However, when you connect with your inner wisdom, the world just looks and feels different, in the best way possible.

I began listening to myself more deeply. What did I want for this moment? This day? This month? What was good in my life, and what did I want to change? What options were available to me for action, and where did it make more sense to wait quietly and see what the universe would do? I started to trust myself, my intuition, and my inner wisdom.

The consistent mindful yoga and meditation practice was an important first step, but I still felt like I wanted to get a deeper level of awareness and understanding of myself. Meditation gave me the ability to observe my present experience, but I felt like I had to do something more, to take action. Perhaps this was my over-striving, problem-solving self running the show.

I knew my mom had used hypnosis for both smoking cessation and weight management, so I thought I'd look into this method of working with your mind. Ever the skeptic and "do-it-myselfer," I began by listening to hypnosis recordings on my own rather than enrolling in one-on-one appointments. After a couple of listening sessions, I noticed I felt safer and more relaxed within my body. There was an open space and lightness inside me where before my brain had felt like a dark, dead-end cave of despair.

The hypnosis was a lot like meditation, but with a goal or task in mind, which satisfied my desire to "do" something. I recognized how hypnotherapy could really help me understand what I wanted for myself in this life, and then take the right actions to get it.

Through hypnosis, I started listening more deeply to my inner wisdom. When I stopped doing/achieving so much and got quieter, this voice of wisdom could become louder and I could start to trust what it told me.

When I practiced the tools I learned in hypnotherapy (which I'll share with you throughout this book so that you can enjoy the results that I have), I finally started feeling like I deserved love simply because I existed, not because of all the things I accomplished. That's still a work in progress to this day, by the way. I still tend to fall into the trap of defining myself by my accomplishments if I don't pay attention. But hypnotherapy allowed me to recognize the state of mind I was aiming for. With this awareness, I can now recognize my safety strategies as they are happening and pause to choose a different action.

My decisions also started to come easier—decisions that were best for me, not for other people. Like saying *no* to that extra PTA meeting that didn't really fit in with my schedule. Or feeling comfortable working outside the home guilt-free instead of staying home with my kids like other people thought I should do. Or taking a yoga class just for me instead of spending an extra hour working.

Recognizing that I subconsciously adopted people-pleasing to feel safe, I suddenly felt empowered to work on new strategies for emotional safety. I stopped saying yes when I really meant no. All of my safety strategies were deeply ingrained in my subconscious behaviors; as with my dependence on accomplishments, I still navigate some of them today. However, when I first became aware of these behaviors and started to transform—what a difference!

I came home with more energy at the end of each week instead of feeling exhausted. I felt joy and peace in my own skin, no matter what I was wearing, how much money I had in the bank, what type of car I drove, what job title I held, or whether or not I'd showered that day.

As I received more glimmers of "Who Sara Is" and started practicing how to authentically align with that Self, I wanted even more. So the next step was to stop trying to guide myself alone and seek out a real expert.

When I went for my first appointment in the hypnotherapist's office, I immediately felt safe and supported in her presence. She radiated a nurturing, disarming energy. I could feel in my body that it was okay to trust her. Her soothing voice and kind nature put me immediately at ease. (Can you think of someone who makes you feel that way? If not, that's okay. You can practice putting yourself at ease first, just like I did.)

As she guided me, I felt at home within myself for possibly the first time ever. I felt safe, I felt secure, I felt like all parts of me were welcome. There was no "bad" or "wrong" part of myself in her office. My whole body dropped into a groove—a "flow"—which allowed for contentment and satisfaction to finally find me. I knew right then this was something I wanted more of. I was hooked.

After a few life-changing sessions with this lovely therapist, my true essence and the life I wanted to lead floated up from the depths of my secret soul to the surface of my being. Then I could inhabit that essence by daily choice instead of keeping it all locked away.

My apathy evaporated more each day. Of course, every life is full of emotions, hardships, losses, and gains. I won't pretend my life is perfect now. But I live out my days by *my* choice. I aim to be as fully present as possible, feeling all the ups and downs gratefully. I nurture the relationships, projects, and directions that feel good to my brain and body, and I don't apologize for who I am.

As I said, those old protective strategies still pop up here and there. But when they do, I am able to quickly recognize what's happening, and then I have a *new* strategy to shift out of protective mode and into alignment. When I do this, it's *glorious*.

Hypnosis allowed me to recognize past limiting beliefs such as "I must fit the status quo to be good enough" and "I must perform and achieve to be loved and not rejected." These beliefs led to unconscious habitual patterns like seeking approval for my decisions, people-pleasing, and biting my tongue instead of speaking my truth. The most difficult part of the journey to change was the recognition of these DNA-deep beliefs. Once I realized that my limiting beliefs governed my behaviors, I could notice when I got stuck in an "undesired" behavior. I could finally start reprogramming the underlying beliefs, and change the way I acted in real life.

In fact, one of the first and most eye-opening facts I learned in my hypnosis training is that approximately 95 percent of our behaviors are driven by our subconscious mind, which houses the beliefs we formed as children! (We will discuss the subconscious mind in more depth in a future chapter.) And when you feel and act differently from the inside, your life inevitably changes on the outside too!

The Evolution of The Mindful Movement

In 2016, my eleven-year-old son suggested I get on YouTube to share my guided meditation and hypnosis recordings so more people could see them. My son helped me set up The Mindful Movement YouTube channel, and I got to work posting videos. It's been a labor of love that I had no idea would be what it is today. The Mindful Movement blew me away with its impact. Today I have an audience of over 895,000 (and growing!) on YouTube, many meditation and hypnosis offerings out in the world, plus a robust list of private hypnotherapy and coaching clients.

While it's wonderful to have a thriving business that supports my family, the best part is that I get to do precisely what my heart most wants—from the deepest part of myself (not the external "stuff" I thought I needed to get to this place). Whenever I witness a client's profound transformations through hypnotherapy, read the comments on the YouTube channel, or hear that my son's English teacher played one of my videos for Mindfulness Monday for the ninth graders, I know I am on the right path!

These life-changing results are also possible for *you*. Let's begin.

Your Turn: Hypnosis

As I have mentioned a few times so far, it is important to trust the process and feel safe enough to allow yourself to receive the benefits available to you. I recommend going to The Mindful Movement YouTube channel and trying a practice or two. You can get to know me, my style, and my voice as a way to get started. There are many different practices to choose from to help you find the right one for you. If you feel called to do so, leave a comment on the video you enjoyed and let me know how you feel after practicing with me.

GO DEEPER REFLECTION QUESTIONS

Keep in mind that you will learn a lot more and have many more opportunities to do your inner work as the book progresses. To begin this process, here are a few reflection questions to consider with curiosity and compassion:

- What experience or behaviors were part of the catalyst for picking up this book?

- What are some behaviors or habits you may have adopted to protect yourself?

- When do you feel most at peace with yourself?

- How can you remind yourself of your inherent worthiness daily?

GO DEEPER AFFIRMATIONS

Here are some affirmations to support your journey with this book. You may choose to write them in your journal and explore how they make you feel when reading them. You can also choose to read them quietly or aloud daily. However you decide to use the affirmations, pay attention to your response to them. How do you feel? What thoughts, images, or memories come up to support or contradict these statements?

- I am enough just as I am, and I embrace my journey with compassion.

- I trust the wisdom within me and believe in my ability to transform my life.

Chapter 2

Getting into the Right State of Mind: How Hypnotherapy Works

My dear intrepid Perfectionist, People Pleaser, Relentless Striver, and Sufferer of imposter syndrome or ADS (Always Doing Something–itis), this chapter is lovingly crafted for *you*. This is for your worrying and questioning part, to satisfy the need for understanding and proof.

Hypnotherapy *works*, and there is so much science behind the magic. You can use self-hypnosis tools or work with a hypnotherapist to gain:

- Improved peace and calm in your body—no more nervous knots in your tummy or tension headaches from stress. You might even reduce your blood pressure!

- An understanding of what may be holding you back from getting what you want in your life.

- The clarity of knowing what drives you, what makes you tick, what lights you up, what your values are, what fulfills and satisfies you from the inside so that you can pursue the life that *you* choose—not live in resentment, exhaustion, depression, resignation, or defeat any longer.

In this pivotal section, we'll dive into how your state of mind enables the power of *suggestion* during hypnosis when you feel safe, supported, relaxed, and nourished. In this state, you can access your emotions and beliefs without the logical part of your mind getting in the way.

"Suggestion" in the context of hypnosis refers to the communication of ideas, thoughts, or commands to the subconscious mind, influencing perceptions, feelings, thoughts, and behaviors. These suggestions can be simple statements or complex visualizations and can impact the subconscious mind profoundly. Suggestions are accepted only if the person believes they are true and possible.

Your Turn: The Power of Suggestion

Close your eyes and imagine holding a bright yellow lemon in your hand. Picture its vibrant color and smooth texture. Now visualize cutting the lemon in half and bringing it up to your nose, inhaling its fresh citrus scent. As you imagine biting into the juicy lemon, feel the tangy juice burst in your mouth, and notice how your body automatically responds.

Likely, this brief activity will cause your mouth to water and your taste buds to tingle. This vivid mental imagery can trigger the physical response or salivation, demonstrating how a simple suggestion can elicit a real, measurable reaction in the body. This is the power of suggestion at work, showing how our thoughts and perceptions can influence our physical state.

Busting a Common Hypnotherapy Myth

Suggestibility is the extent to which a person is able to accept and act on suggestions given during hypnosis. It is a natural and normal phenomenon that varies from person to person. Some individuals are more suggestible than others, which means they can easily enter a state of heightened focus and receptivity, making them more responsive to hypnotic suggestions.

During hypnosis, the conscious mind becomes less critical and analytical, allowing the subconscious mind to be more open to suggestions. One common misconception about hypnosis is that it involves a loss of control or that the hypnotist can make the individual do things against their will. You may think that during hypnosis, you will be out of control and do something you don't want to do or adopt beliefs and values that are not true to you or your character. In reality, hypnotherapy is a collaborative process. The individual remains fully aware and in control throughout the session. In hypnosis, you are in complete control, and your mind will show you only what you are ready to understand. You will plant the seeds for only the new beliefs you want to have.

Before we continue with the science, let me add that the changes you wish to see will still take discovery, reflection, and action. It's not like you'll leave a hypnosis session with a totally new identity and then turn your life upside down.

Though most of my clients *do* report feeling lighter, calmer, less anxious, and more grounded after each session, changes continue to happen days, weeks, and months after we meet. I provide all my clients with a personalized hypnosis recording to listen to daily so that they reinforce the mindset and belief changes they've made during the primary session. As you will learn, the mind loves what is familiar, so you will need to make your new beliefs familiar with consistent practice.

I cannot emphasize enough that this therapeutic modality is always under your control. Though the goal of hypnotherapy is to open you up to safe and courageous suggestibility, you still maintain awareness and choice throughout the entire process. Your mind will not allow you to push harder than you can handle—you'll always be in charge of the pace and the depth of the inner work and how you behave afterward.

So let's uncover how your brain and suggestibility work together!

Brain Wave States and Hypnosis

Hmmmm, what actually *is* hypnosis?

The Mayo Clinic says it's "a changed state of awareness and increased relaxation that allows for improved focus and concentration."

And the all-knowing Merriam-Webster says it's "a trancelike state of altered consciousness that resembles sleep but is induced by a person whose suggestions are readily accepted by the subject."

In truth, we've *all* experienced a trancelike state without any outside help from a hypnotherapist. If you've ever allowed a parent, teacher, peer, politician, religious leader, news outlet, or social media channel or account to suggest a thought, mindset, action, or concept to you, you've experienced a very mild form of hypnosis.

Notice how you tend to let in the suggestions that feel safe, familiar, and keep your values. For example, we can be influenced into the action by a loved one's advice about our lives.

Here's another fun way to discover how a trancelike state can come about in your regular waking life. Have you ever:

- Bought something you later realized you didn't want?
- Driven home, only to realize you don't remember the last four turns you made?

- Felt the emotions of the characters on TV or in a movie?

When you're in this trance-like state, it means that your subconscious brain is a tad more in the driver's seat of your life. And it's the subconscious brain that we really want to bring to the surface during hypnotherapy.

With all that being said, you will *never* accept any suggestions under hypnosis that you don't agree with or believe in when you're fully conscious.

Your Amazing Subconscious Brain

You know that old saying that we use only about 10 percent of our brains? While that's not at all accurate—every cell in our brain has an active role to play in our lives—it's fair to say that only approximately 5 percent of our actions are driven by our conscious minds. This is useful because it would be exhausting to have to consciously take every action we make. Think about all of the actions you take without consciously thinking about them when you drive a car, for example.

The conscious mind is like the tip of the iceberg that is visible above the surface of the ocean. Everything below the surface represents your subconscious mind.

Your conscious brain does the following:

- Makes your daily decisions, like choosing the quickest way to get to work while avoiding big traffic jams.
- Works on the "reality" principle—always grounded in what is, not what could be.
- Uses logic exclusively, not imagination or intuition.
- Provides practical analysis. (How high is that curb I have to step off of? Can I cross the street before that bus

down the road hits me? Which color shirt will go best with these pants?)

- Reasons out possible outcomes for decisions you make, based on an understanding of cause and effect. (If "A," then "B.")

- Enjoys a negativity bias, which means preparing for the worst possible outcome of any situation.

- Stores short-term memories, like remembering what you said to your friend five minutes ago so you don't repeat yourself.

Your subconscious brain, on the other hand, guides your life in this way:

- Implements all of your autopilot processes like driving, using utensils, or typing on the computer.

- Takes everything literally from the conscious mind. (For example, if you use the word "my" in front of a diagnosis, such as "my anxiety," the mind believes you are taking ownership of it and want to keep it. The alternative is "the anxiety," which sends a message that it is not yours and you don't want to keep it. Consider this when comparing "my husband" vs. "the husband.")

- Will do exactly what the conscious mind focuses on. (For example, if you are always worrying about failing your presentation for work, then you'll likely choke on "game day." What you focus on, you attract. If you were told not to think about a pink elephant, you would first think about that pink elephant in order to know what *not* to think about.)

- Does what it thinks you want it to do. An example of this is when your narrative is "this job is killing me," and then you mysteriously come down with the flu and have to take a week off of work. While the mind doesn't "cause" the flu (a virus would), you open yourself up for illness with this type of thinking, and you may be more susceptible.

- Moves toward pleasure, away from pain, instinctively. (Dependent on your definitions of pleasurable and painful, examples might be moving toward that extra doughnut, toward another round of satisfying sex, or away from the uncomfortable conversation with your partner or boss.)

- Moves toward the familiar, away from the unfamiliar (even if the familiar is troubling, challenging, or harmful to yourself or others).

- Responds to words and pictures you offer yourself by giving you visceral sensations or emotions (like when your mouth waters if you think about ice cream, or when your heart races if you think about your latest crush).

A hypnotherapy session allows your conscious mind to relax and feel safe enough to move aside so that the subconscious mind can take center stage. By interacting with your subconscious more directly, you'll be able to discover past messaging and inner beliefs that could be holding you hostage to your current coping behaviors.

In other words, the anxiety, the people-pleasing, the perfectionism, the over-striving, the unending comparison and self-judgment all have roots in your subconscious mind. Hypnotherapy is one effective way of getting your conscious, analytical brain to move aside long enough so that the foundation of your struggle can come to the surface to be healed, morphed, and gently remodeled without abruptness or fear.

Getting Out of Fight, Flight, Fawn, or Freeze Mode

The nervous system is complex and has a big role in how we experience life. For the purpose of this book, I'll share a very basic introduction to how it works to help you understand the way your nervous system may be contributing to your experience and how you can use it to support you. For more depth on the topic, refer to the resources at the end of this book.

Many of us have heard about fight-or-flight mode. Perhaps you know the analogy describing what happens when a bear chases us in the woods. Our bodies leap into action without thought and we run away with the strength and speed of an Olympian. Or if we're backed into a corner, we make ourselves as big and scary as we can. In these moments, all our senses are on hyperalert and we have more strength than we ever imagined possible. Our nonessential bodily functions shut down to divert all of our energy to survival.

But what about "fawn"? This is a lesser-known trick of your nervous system to placate, submit, or acquiesce our way back into safety from a place of danger when that's the quickest way back to homeostasis. A prime example of this fawn response could take the shape of very skillful flattery or an overabundant nurturing in relationships to avoid conflict, abuse, or abandonment.

The freeze response is your brain's go-to resource when all else fails—it's a total shutdown. Your thinking, logical brain is completely offline, and in this state, you're simply trying not to die, so you surrender and go limp or even leave your body and go somewhere else safer in your mind. This is the equivalent of an animal playing dead to protect itself from a predator.

Here are some ways that your fight/flight/freeze/fawn response may show up in real life:

- Working fifteen-hour days for weeks on end to prove yourself and your worth through accomplishments (fight response)

- Using substances, shopping, or food to "take the edge off" at the end of the day (flight or freeze)

- Getting defensive when receiving constructive feedback at work (fight)

- Watching TV for hours on end (freeze)

- Startling easily (flight)

- Experiencing tension in your shoulders and a clenched jaw (fight)

- Losing your sense of self (fawn)

If a lot of your waking hours are spent in a mild or dramatic activation of fight-or-flight mode, your *sympathetic nervous system* is stuck in the "on" position. When this "survival" portion of our brain lights up, we cannot take on anything new. Learning becomes impossible, because all we can focus on is how to survive the next several minutes without dying, even if you're not in any real imminent danger. Remember, nonessential functions, like digestion or reproductive hormone activity, shut down when you are in survival mode.

Those of you who feel continual stomach butterflies, shoulder tension, or a racing mind (chock-full of your packed to-do list and the resulting guilt or inadequacy of not completing every task) know well the toll your sympathetic nervous system can take on you when it's always running the show.

The *opposite* of the fight-or-flight response is your rest-and-digest mode, or *parasympathetic nervous system*. This is the system that we need to come online for learning, integration, change, adopting new behaviors, or embracing novel self-awareness and inner evolution. It is also the system we need for healing and digestion. You know you're operating within your parasympathetic nervous system when:

- Your gut feels calm and relaxed—not too empty and not too full, not churning with stress and anxiety.
- Your muscles feel calm and loose—your shoulders sit comfortably, far away from your ears.
- Your jaw loosens up.
- Your teeth stop clenching.
- Your tension headache disappears.
- Your thoughts feel spacious and even a little wandering—there are no obsessive or intrusive threads upon which to fixate.
- You can think clearly and learn something new.

The Nervous System in Action

As a hypnotherapist, I had the pleasure of working with Daniel, a thirty-five-year-old corporate executive struggling with increasing stress and anxiety. Daniel had always prided himself on his resilience, but recently, even minor inconveniences left him feeling overwhelmed.

During our work together, Daniel described a typical stressful event: being stuck in traffic while running late for an important meeting. He noted his heart pounding, a tightness in his chest, and clammy hands. I explained how these physical symptoms were signs of his sympathetic nervous system activating a fight-or-flight response.

To help Daniel manage these responses, I guided him through a visualization exercise. He recalled the stressful event, noticing his physical sensations. I then introduced techniques he could use to activate his parasympathetic nervous system, such as deep breathing, gently rubbing his arms, and grounding techniques like feeling his feet on the floor.

Over the next few weeks, Daniel practiced being aware of the activation of the stress response and then using these calming techniques regularly. He became more aware of his body's stress signals and learned to intervene before his anxiety escalated. This increased awareness and use of calming strategies helped Daniel feel more in control and resilient. Daniel was able to increase both his capacity to hold stress and his ability to regulate his unique nervous system.

Daniel's experience demonstrates how understanding your own specific nervous system reactions in stress responses can empower you to manage your stress effectively and improve overall well-being.

Your Turn: Activate Your Parasympathetic Nervous System State

Switching on your parasympathetic nervous system may require some practice, especially if you're wired up for the apocalypse most of the time. Try it now! Slow down and take several long, slow, intentional breaths. As you breathe, focus on making your exhales longer and slower.

If you really were in danger, you wouldn't be able to slow your breath down. The fact that you *can* have this control over your breathing sends a message to your nervous system that you're really not in peril. Take a moment to experiment.

If it is helpful, you can count the length of your inhale, and make your exhale twice as long. For example, if your inhale takes three counts, try to make your exhale six counts.

Did you do it? How does your body feel? My hope for you is that every time you try a relaxation practice, you might notice a little more spaciousness and calm in your body and brain. The two sides of your nervous system can and should work together to keep you out of relentless survival mode. When you really need that system—like when you're *actually* being chased by a bear—it'll still be available to you. But it's time to stop *feeling* like a bear is chasing you every day.

You could also add some gentle rocking or a self-hug, like you would soothe a child or baby. Another good practice for parasympathetic turn-on is to slow down your eating a bit, especially if you typically rush right through each meal. Taking time to taste, chew, and swallow your food, even just for *one* meal each day, is an effective way to get your rest-and-digest mojo flowing more reliably. Again, when you are in survival mode, digestion gets turned off because all your inner resources get diverted to outrunning the bear.

As you begin to explore hypnosis and some of the activities in this book, you will get to know your personal nervous system signals. You will begin to use this information to recognize when you unconsciously move into survival mode. The activity at the end of this chapter will help you create a road map of your nervous system patterns so that you can more quickly drop into ease.

Bonus: I offer loads of free resources for easy, short meditations and relaxation tools on my YouTube channel, The Mindful Movement, many of which are designed to keep your parasympathetic nervous system in the driver's seat.

Brainwave States and the Subconscious Mind

Once we have strong access to our parasympathetic nervous system within a hypnosis session, the subconscious mind becomes more accessible. That's where the results and "ahas" happen.

Your mind has these four states of being:

- Beta, where we experience normal waking states of consciousness
- Alpha, whose job is relaxation, visualization, and creativity
- Theta, which is responsible for meditation, intuition, and memory
- Delta, which gives us detached awareness, healing, and sleep

Your *Beta*, or conscious, state is where you're most aware of your physical senses to receive input and information from the world around you so that you can respond in the moment to keep yourself fed, sheltered, productive, and safe. If you're spending too much time in this brainstate relative to the other three states, you could struggle with:

- Higher blood pressure
- Muscle tension
- Anxiety
- Aggression

When this brainstate is in balance with the other three states, you are alert, engaged, discerning, focused, and able to make confident decisions plus complete tasks quickly and adeptly. A few examples of classic Beta activities include:

- Taking exams
- Playing sports
- Giving presentations
- Engaging in conversation
- Cooking an intricate recipe

The *Alpha* state is where we get to do a lot of creative and satisfying tasks, like:

- Relaxing our minds and bodies
- Visualizing or conceptualizing different desires, pathways, or outcomes
- Finding resonance with the earth's frequency (yes, that's a thing)
- Relieving stress and anxiety

The Alpha state is also the gateway to deeper states of consciousness—where we can "ideate" and explore new ways of being within ourselves that feel more welcoming, forgiving, and secure; relate with others; and move toward the goals our conscious mind desires! Classic Alpha activities include:

- Going with the flow
- Relaxing in a comfy chair or on a mat or couch
- Receiving inspiration
- Exploring your creativity
- Learning from a source you love
- Developing your inner consciousness—how you "work" and feel from the inside out

Your *Theta* state helps you:

- Meditate (quiet your thoughts and enjoy inner focus plus a calmer state of being)

- Access your intuition (the subtle nudges and "gut" feelings that can offer synchronistic experiences and happy or well-timed outcomes)

- Review memories and gain insight from them

Your *Theta* state feels like waking dreams complete with vivid imagery, plus being receptive to information beyond normal conscious awareness, as if the universe had a direct "download" to your brain and heart. The Theta state is where many people experience the utter bliss and soul-unity of deep meditation, as well as accessing blocked memories that can offer insight into why you're stuck in the present day, or where your intrinsic messaging and self-beliefs originated. Theta activities include:

- The moments right before sleep

- Deep meditation

- Super-learning (think "downloads" from the universe)

- Dream recall

- Self-hypnosis

- Recovery of lost memories

The *Delta* state is where you do your deepest sleep, detachment, and recovery. This state is crucial for healing and bodily homeostasis. You definitely know it if you haven't visited this state in a while. None of our physical or mental systems can function optimally without spending seven to nine hours per night in this supremely healing brainstate. Hallmark activities of the Delta state include:

- Having detached awareness
- Healing
- Sleeping
- Very deep sleeping, being unconscious

Delta state activities center around bodily healing and recovery. You might know you're in the Delta state sweet spot if you enjoy:

- Healing ability
- Controlled blood pressure and heart rate
- Low muscle tension
- Improved digestion

If you've ever fallen asleep chewing on a problem and woken up in the morning with just the solution you need, you've likely enjoyed some productive Delta state time. Dropping into very deep sleep, noticing better learning and recall, feeling your intuition get "louder," and having greater peace of mind are all benefits of this brainstate.

YOUR TURN:
CREATE A NERVOUS SYSTEM ROAD MAP

In order to build resilience and have more control to make shifts in your nervous system, it is important to get to know your unique nervous system. All humans respond differently to stress and in this activity, you can get to know your personal stress response tendencies. This will help you to recognize stress in your body so you can regulate your nervous system when needed.

Step 1: Recall a Stressful Event

Call to mind a recent stressful event. Aim for something that you might categorize as a 3 or 4 on a scale of 1–10, with 10 being the most stressful. You can work through this process in your mind or grab your journal and jot some things down.

Step 2: Observe Physical Responses

When you think of this event, what do you remember feeling in your body? As you recall the event in the present, what do you notice in your body now? Reflect on the following:

- Heart Rate: Do you sense an increase in your heart rate?

- Temperature: Is there an increase in your body temperature?

- Tension: Do you notice any tightness or clenching in your muscles?

These responses are your body's natural reactions to stress. Everyone's reactions can differ, and it's helpful to recognize your unique patterns.

Step 3: Practice Self-Soothing and Grounding

After noticing these reactions, shift your focus to calming techniques:

- Extended Exhales: Practice taking deep breaths with a focus on lengthening the exhale.
- Self-Soothing Strategies: Engage in gentle actions such as rubbing your arms or legs, rocking, or placing a hand on areas of tightness.
- Grounding Techniques: Use techniques that help you feel more connected to the present moment and your surroundings.

Step 4: Develop Your Tool Kit

With practice, you can develop a personalized list of go-to strategies that effectively calm your nervous system. Reflect on which techniques work best for you and note them down. Over time, you will be able to:

- Recognize patterns of stress activation in your body.
- Identify and use tools or methods that help you calm down.
- Build resilience by regularly practicing these calming techniques.

By understanding and mapping your nervous system's responses, you empower yourself to manage stress more effectively and foster a greater sense of well-being.

GO DEEPER REFLECTION QUESTIONS

- How does your body typically respond to stress?
- Which self-soothing or grounding techniques have you found most effective in calming your nervous system?
- In what ways can you incorporate these calming strategies into your daily routine to build resilience against stress?

GO DEEPER AFFIRMATIONS

- I am aware of my body's responses to stress, and I accept them with compassion and understanding.
- Each time I practice calming my nervous system, I build resilience and strengthen my ability to handle stress.

With a greater understanding of the mind's four states and how they work, you can apply this knowledge to your present situation and what you'd like to change in hypnotherapy. Change begins with uncovering an issue that's holding you back, because change can't come without awareness first.

It's time to uncover your specific issue in the intake process. Let's go.

Chapter 3

Getting Started with Hypnotherapy

Before step 1, the intake, can even begin, the client has to recognize that there is an aspect of their life they want to improve or change, and that they need support in doing so. Here's a fun fact: When you try to change yourself without a coach, helper, professional, or guide, it's like trying to get a clear picture of yourself with your nose pressed against a mirror. It's blurry, distorted, and probably not your best angle. The hypnotherapist's job is to pull the mirror back so that you can see more clearly what you'd like to keep and what needs to shift.

You can also compare going it alone to trying to fix a car without opening the hood to see the engine. How will you know if the issue is the alternator or the transmission? You're pretty likely to waste time, effort, and money when you cannot clearly define the issue because you're too close to it or cannot see what's going on.

By picking up this book, you've already opened yourself up to a collaboration. You and I are working together to allow you to understand yourself better and to facilitate the changes you wish to make in your life. The previous chapters set the stage for understanding the importance of the intake process, where we gather vital information that will help guide your journey toward personal growth and transformation.

If you were my client, you would start with a thorough reflection process before we would even begin any hypnosis. There are several questions I ask that are crucial to a successful hypnosis experience. These powerful questions provide a tool to allow you to see what you couldn't see about yourself before. And remember, you can't change what you don't first acknowledge and accept.

My clients often tell me I have asked a question they never considered, which gave them a whole new lens on their main issue or challenge. Or the answer to the questions might connect some dots, showing you how the past has influenced the present—which may never have occurred to you before.

People are often surprised by how much comes up during the process of completing this intake form, and continues to come to the surface before the session. The "work" of hypnosis begins even before the client's first appointment.

Think back to when you bought this book. With that action, you already became ready to entertain a transformation for yourself. The simple act of buying the book created a container for change. You may have noticed memories of your past surfacing, dreams for your life taking clearer shape, or even unexplained emotions coming up seemingly out of the blue.

Maybe you even resisted getting started reading, because reading would mean you'd have to look more deeply at yourself and feel uncomfortable or even disturbing feelings. Your old pattern of procrastination may come up with a vengeance, even as you consider living your life in a different way. Almost like a form of rebellion, this voice may surface with a message: "Oh, you think you're really going to change? Who do you think you are, anyway?"

Think about it—if you've ever embarked on a diet that restricted *all* chocolate, maybe you ate a *lot* of chocolate the day before your new diet was set to begin. Guess what? Resistance to change is completely natural. You should expect it as you move through this book. As you'll discover in detail in just a few pages, one of the Principles of the Mind is to avoid discomfort and anything unfamiliar. The good news is that with hypnotherapy, you can begin to understand and befriend your mind's resistance to growth and change.

When you are safe—when your nervous system senses safety—you have all the answers to your deep and curious questions. You are free to uncover the places that you've protected for a *long* time out of fear, which turns into habit over time. So when I ask an intake question and you answer, "I don't know," you probably really do know.

INTAKE IN ACTION

Ashlyn, a successful entrepreneur, found herself drowning in overwhelm and burnout. Despite her accomplishments, she was constantly stressed, feeling like she was on a never-ending treadmill. She noticed that her days were filled with tasks she didn't want to do and that didn't contribute to her business growth. Her inability to say no led her to take on more work than she could handle. She felt an intense need to do everything herself, believing that no one else could meet her standards.

Ashlyn's people-pleasing behaviors and hyper-responsibility were evident. At work, she was the go-to person for everyone, always ready to help her colleagues, often at the expense of her own projects. She was the last to leave the office, staying late to finish tasks that could have been delegated. She rarely took breaks, driven by an internal voice telling her she needed to prove her worth through hard work and dedication.

At home, the pattern continued. Ashlyn managed everything, from household chores to organizing family events. She felt responsible for her family's well-being and often sacrificed her own needs to ensure their happiness. The constant pressure to be perfect and meet everyone's expectations left her exhausted and resentful.

The turning point came when Ashlyn decided to seek hypnotherapy. As she completed the intake questionnaire, she began to reflect deeply on her past and her relationships with her primary caretakers. The questions prompted her to consider how her childhood experiences shaped her current behaviors.

Ashlyn grew up with a single mom who relied heavily on her to take on adult responsibilities. From a young age, Ashlyn learned to prioritize her mother's needs over her own. Her mom's wants always came first, and Ashlyn's needs were often overlooked. This dynamic instilled in her a belief that her worth was tied to how well she could serve others and handle responsibilities.

As Ashlyn answered the questions on the intake form, she started connecting the dots. She realized that her inability to delegate and her tendency to overcommit were rooted in her childhood experiences. The hyper-responsibility and people-pleasing behaviors were survival strategies she had developed to cope with her early environment. Recognizing this pattern was a pivotal moment for her.

Armed with this new awareness, Ashlyn began to take baby steps toward change. She started setting boundaries at work, learning to say no to tasks that didn't align with her goals. She delegated responsibilities and trusted her team more, which not only reduced her workload but also empowered her colleagues. At home, she practiced self-care, allowing herself to relax and prioritize her own needs.

The intake process provided Ashlyn with significant insights even before her hypnotherapy session. This initial self-reflection set the stage for her therapeutic journey, giving her a clearer understanding of her patterns and the origins of her stress. As a result, Ashlyn felt more prepared and motivated to engage in the hypnotherapy process, knowing that she was already making progress in understanding and addressing her challenges.

Ashlyn's story illustrates the transformative power of the intake process. By answering deep, thoughtful questions, she uncovered the roots of her overwhelm and burnout. This preliminary work not only provided immediate value but also laid a strong foundation for the transformative journey ahead. Through hypnotherapy, Ashlyn continued to build on these insights, ultimately achieving a more balanced and fulfilling life.

Powerful Questions, Powerful Results

The process of reflection when completing the intake form provided Ashlyn with several benefits:

- Self-Reflection: By thoughtfully answering the intake questions, Ashlyn started to reflect on her life and behaviors, gaining deeper insight into her patterns.

- Opportunity to Connect Past to Present: She was able to link her childhood experiences to her current tendencies, understanding how her past shaped her present actions.

- Increased Awareness: This new awareness enabled her to see that her reluctance to delegate and her tendency to overcommit were rooted in old survival strategies.

- Empowerment for Change: Recognizing these patterns allowed Ashlyn to feel empowered to start making small, meaningful changes in her life and business.

The intake process serves as a powerful tool, setting the stage for effective hypnotherapy by uncovering important insights and fostering self-awareness even before the first session. This preparatory work helps clients like Ashlyn gain clarity and begin their journey of transformation with a solid understanding of the underlying issues they want to address.

YOUR TURN: INTAKE

Take a moment to reflect on what brought you to this book in the first place. Answer the following reflection questions as if you were preparing for a personalized hypnotherapy session. Take your time and go deep with your answers. Don't just brush the surface. If it gets a little intense, put down the book, take a walk, call a friend, or do something nourishing for yourself.

GO DEEPER REFLECTION QUESTIONS

- How has the presenting issue that brought you to this book served you, protected you, or helped you so far in your life?

We don't do things that don't serve us in some way, even if they aren't desirable or logical.

- What have you made this issue, symptom, or behavior mean about you?

  We naturally tell ourselves stories about the events, feelings, challenges, or triumphs in our lives to make them mean something—we are meaning makers at our core.

- What is the underlying unmet need?

  Most issues come down to a gap we feel between our reality and our desires for approval, control, security, connection, and love.

- What does it cost you to stay the same and stuck?

  We often keep doing the same thing because it is more comfortable to do what's familiar, even if it isn't what we really want or what is best for us.

- What are some of the labels you have given yourself, or been given by others, in your life?

  Labels go deeper than Wife, Husband, Mother, Student, or Employee. They can also look like Failure, Screwup, Slob, Flake, Angel, Nerd, Jock, or the Perfect Child.

- What are the beliefs that you developed about yourself as a child?

  These beliefs could sound like "I have to be pretty all the time," or "I can help my parents feel better," or even "I never win at anything, so I'll just sit out instead."

- What are some of the behaviors you feel are "part of your personality," but could really be a safety strategy?

These are the areas that *could change* and make your life better, even if they are so familiar it's hard to let them go or picture yourself without that piece of your identity.

YOUR TURN:
BUILDING CONNECTION TO INNER WISDOM

Try this simple exercise to dip your toe into the world of hypnotherapy. Begin by making yourself comfortable in a safe and supported posture. (Safety is important to make sure you are in a learning state, rather than fight-or-flight.) It's fine to sit in a comfortable chair or on the floor. Close your eyes if you like.

Take a few long, slow breaths in through your nose and out through your mouth. Once settled, let go of any effort related to your breathing. Allow your breath to be effortless and nourishing.

Connect with your true essence or your Self energy. This is the *you* that is compassionate, curious, and confident of your worth. This is the *you* that feels safe and is pure awareness. You may have a sense of spaciousness and at the same time connectedness. You may notice a buzzing or vibrating energy that is your Self energy. Be with this experience for a moment.

From a place of your true essence, ask that this exercise be in support of and in alignment with your highest good. Know that your mind wants what is best for you and will only bring to the surface what you are ready and able to understand.

With curiosity and compassion for yourself, go through the following inquiry process and give yourself some time to allow the experience to unfold organically and your inner wisdom to come to the surface without thinking or trying.

Notice the most prominent sensation in your body right now. Be with the sensation, breathe into the sensation. Imagine all of the pores of your skin have the ability to breathe and send your inhale directly into the sensation you are experiencing. Where is this sensation located in your body? How does it feel? (Painful, easeful, uncomfortable, tense, relaxed, or something else?)

Continue to stay with the sensation and consider, What does this sensation need from you? Does this sensation have a message for you? A nudge of recognition? Or some inner wisdom?

What else in your body needs your attention most right now? Be with this part of you. Take a few long, slow breaths. Relax and connect even more deeply with yourself. If emotions come up, allow them to move through you without restriction. Know that emotions are energy in motion and you can allow them to be in motion so they aren't pushed down or recycled.

Are there any messages or anything this other part of you wants you to know? Sit with the information that comes. Relax and soften your body and mind.

Let go of thinking and trying, and allow yourself to have the experience naturally. You are on a journey of information, and this is just the beginning. There is nothing you have to solve or act upon right now. It's okay to remain in this relaxed and deep state for as long as you like, as long as messages keep coming through for you. There are no wrong answers or silly messages. This is simply your body and your subconscious communicating with you.

When you feel complete, thank yourself, thank your body, thank your mind, and thank all the information you have received. Come back to full awareness gradually and take time to write down some of the key information that came to you out of this experience.

Feel free to journal more extensively about what you learned or came away with during this exercise, as it will be essential moving forward.

GO DEEPER AFFIRMATIONS

- I trust my inner wisdom and allow it to guide me toward my highest good.
- My mind and body are aligned, and I am open to receiving the messages they share.
- I approach myself with curiosity and compassion, honoring my journey and experiences.

Remember, all we do in the intake process is increase our whole-person awareness. There is no other action to take, nothing to "fix." Just connect deeply and willingly with your brain and body. You can trust them both.

Our next step is making sense of our intake responses with a deeper understanding of the Principles of the Mind.

Chapter 4

Principles of the Mind

Many of my clients come to see me because they cannot quite figure out how they got so stuck in their lives. Even if they can *see* their misaligned or destructive behaviors, they can't help but wonder why they still cannot seem to change them.

My clients will talk about relationships that falter because of their workaholism or perfectionism. Some are continually chasing the next shiny outfit, vacation, or SUV in hope of fulfillment and contentment. Others are getting so burned out at work that they keep getting sick, feel exhausted all the time, and can't remember their last happy moment.

I mean, it should be *easy*, right? If you understand how your life isn't going as you planned or wanted, then you should be able to course-correct into different actions that get you on track for the joy, satisfaction, contentment, and peace you've so deeply desired.

I hate being the bearer of bad news, but our brains don't work that way. Otherwise, there would be no anxiety, stress, people-pleasing, or toxic striving. I would be out of a job if the awareness of an issue or undesired experience was all that was needed to change it.

At the foundation of hypnotherapy are several principles that the mind follows without our even being conscious of them. Even when we notice areas of our lives we want to change, these rules generally steer the mind toward the status quo. This can make it super challenging to make lasting changes in behavior. *Argh*, right?

These principles have evolved over time, influenced by the contributions of key figures such as Milton Erickson, Charles Tebbetts, Franz Mesmer, James Braid, Jean-Martin Charcot, and Dave Elman, among others. The Principles of the Mind are evidence based (which means you can scientifically test them for repeatability and predictability) and can help us communicate with the subconscious mind more effectively for true inner and outer transformation.

Unless you know how the mind works, you'll likely self-sabotage your attempts at change—because your brain really likes what it knows and will do everything it can to get back to the familiar, even if the "familiar" is painful, miserable, or destructive. We always look for confirmation from the world that our beliefs about it are true and reliable.

Here's a basic tutorial on the Principles of the Mind so you can begin to see how they play out in your life.

Every Thought or Idea Causes a Physical Reaction

What happens in your body when you get angry? If you're like many people, your blood pressure may rise, your breathing may quicken, and you may start sweating or feeling jumpy in your skin. When you're sad, you may want to crumble into a ball under a blanket, cry your eyes out, or even numb out and go to sleep. When you feel inspired by a new idea, you may want to walk or run off some of that big energy or grab a sheet of paper and some art supplies so you can get your idea out where you can see it.

You likely have a go-to set of actions or physical sensations when you feel a strong emotion. These responses became part of your "normal" when you were a child or young adult. A classic example here is a parent who says (or yells), "I'll give you something to cry about!" when their child gets upset. That child may develop a lifelong conditioned response of bodily shutdown in response to their strong emotions—because it wasn't safe to have them at home.

Another classic and relatable example is public speaking. Imagine you're about to give a public speech. The mere thought of speaking in front of an audience can make your heart race, palms sweat, and stomach churn, even though you haven't started speaking yet. As a child, you might have experienced ridicule or criticism from a harsh teacher or critical classmates when speaking in front of others. This early negative experience created a strong association between public speaking and fear, causing physical anxiety symptoms when you think about speaking publicly.

Whatever your own childhood experience, your body has become conditioned to respond in certain ways to strong emotions over time. If you want to change these physical responses to your emotions, you must reach them at the place where they began.

What You Expect, You Experience

Your brain and nerves respond to images, either real or imagined. This means that even if you conjure up a scene in your mind based on nothing but fantasy, your body will respond to it and experience all the sensations as if that scene were happening in real life. Additionally, your body remembers your brain's mental images and the corresponding physical responses even if your mind doesn't consciously remember. People will often refer to this as being "triggered" or "activated."

If you constantly worry about failing a test, you might start to believe you will fail, which can increase anxiety and affect your performance negatively. Growing up, you may have had overly critical parents who focused on your mistakes and failures, leading you to develop a negative expectancy around your abilities. This ingrained belief makes you prone to anxiety and poor performance in situations where you anticipate failure.

Your Mind Moves You Toward Pleasure and Away from Pain (Based on How You Define Them)

Your mind subconsciously leads you toward what is pleasurable based on your definition of pleasure. This means that you must very carefully look at what is pleasurable and painful to you about your behavior. There is always some kind of payoff in the behaviors we repeat even if we know they are unhealthy, unhelpful, or even destructive.

Consider this example. You know that you are qualified and ready for a promotion at work (which will get you closer to your dream house, a more flexible schedule, and increased leadership impact and influence), but you must speak up and apply to be considered. However, you got the message very early on from your immigrant parents that failure and mistakes are not okay. They always told you it's better to stay quiet and invisible to get along in the world so that you don't risk messing up.

Because of this deep belief handed down to you, you do *not* apply for the promotion. The fear of failure and the accompanying terror of so much visibility feel too big for you to handle. So you languish in your current role in order to stay "safe" and "comfortable" at all costs.

Until you change this inner messaging about what it means to get along in your world, your brain will scramble at every turn to stay invisible, small, and "safe." And even though small and safe feel miserable to you, the alternative risk of visibility, impact, and potential failure are even worse, if only in the short term.

Your brain will always choose the more pleasurable of two options, even if they are both less than ideal. In the previous example, it's less painful and more familiar to stay small and safe, and more painful to risk failure. Until you can change the *root* of what your brain defines as pleasurable or painful, you'll always move toward what your subconscious mind believes is the safer option.

Carin's story is a clear example of this principle. When Carin was a little girl, the message she received from her parents was that she was to be seen and not heard. She understood that her needs and emotions were not important. Now that she is an adult, when she has an argument with her husband, she shuts down, gets very quiet and submissive, and never says what is most important to her. She senses that he is upset and her little girl inside is reactivated. It's as if she goes back in time and becomes the little girl who believes it is safer for her to hide herself, make herself small, and keep her voice inside. This shutdown makes her husband even more upset because he believes she is ignoring him or rejecting him, which perpetuates the cycle even more.

Your Mind Moves You Toward the Familiar and Away from the Unfamiliar (Even If the Familiar Is Hurtful, Damaging, or Uncomfortable)

We've *all* experienced this principle. We can all look within and come up with a time we chose a familiar action over the one that would've best served us, like choosing the same type of emotionally unavailable partner time and time again. You know this person is not good for you and will not love you in the way you really want to be loved. But you cannot feel any attraction toward someone different and likely better for you.

Here's another powerful demonstration of this principle at work. Laura was the youngest of seven siblings and grew up with emotionally unavailable, strict parents. She is currently in a conflict with her boss at work. If there was conflict or disagreements in her family growing up, her parents were always right and their way was the only way, no matter what. This was so familiar to her as the youngest child, she didn't know any other way. Now she is having a hard time standing up for herself and speaking her values. Even though she knows that speaking her mind is important for her career, it is so unfamiliar and unsafe that she cannot do what she knows she needs to do.

Opposing Ideas Cannot Be Held Simultaneously

If what you think and believe on the inside aren't the same as how you behave on the outside, your body, relationships, finances, and life path will reap the consequences. This means that your brain will subconsciously do everything it can to ensure that your actions match your beliefs—even if your conscious mind knows that your current behavior patterns are hurting you. When you see this process in your own life, it's a huge clue that your inner messaging needs a tune-up first. Only when you change your inner beliefs can your outer behavior change to match what you tell yourself on the inside.

Thirty-seven-year-old Megan's biggest desire in life was to get married and have a family. Yet she continued to create conflicts in any long-term relationships she had. She usually ended any potential relationship by very quickly finding a variety of reasons why the men she dated weren't right for her.

Megan had the subconscious belief that she was unlovable. Her father was never part of her life. Her mother was seventeen when she was born, so her grandparents raised her. Although Megan's grandparents loved her and did the best they could raising her, Megan believed she was unlovable and this is why her parents "abandoned" her. This underlying belief was driving her current relationship behaviors and sabotaging her partnerships before they got off the ground, even though what she wanted most of all was to be loved.

Megan first needed to change her internal beliefs in order to change her external behaviors in her relationships.

Once an Idea Is Accepted by the Subconscious, It Remains Until Replaced

Megan from the previous story is a clear example of one belief remaining until it is replaced with another. The idea that she was unlovable drove all of her actions in her dating life until Megan replaced it with the idea that she was lovable.

A person who grew up believing they're not good at math might continue to struggle with math-related tasks as an adult, despite new learning opportunities, because the old belief remains until actively replaced with a new, positive belief. In school, if a teacher or parent repeatedly told you that you were bad at math, this negative belief could have taken root in your subconscious. Despite later success or opportunities to learn, the old belief persists until it's consciously addressed and changed.

Your Mind Always Listens and Responds to What You Tell Yourself

Your mind is always attuned to your internal dialogue and responds to the words and thoughts you repeatedly affirm. This principle underscores the importance of maintaining positive and constructive self-talk because what you tell yourself shapes your reality and influences your mental and physical states.

This rule shows up in the self-protecting behaviors you find yourself doing often but don't consciously choose. Here are some examples of habitual behaviors and the deeper impulses that might underlie them.

Emma has always dreaded public speaking. Whenever she has to present at work, she tells herself, "I'm going to mess up. Everyone will see how nervous I am." As Emma repeats these thoughts, her body reacts with increased heart rate, sweating, and a shaky voice. These physical symptoms reinforce her belief that she's a poor public speaker, making each experience more anxiety inducing than the last.

Emma's self-talk about failing at public speaking creates a self-fulfilling prophecy. Her mind listens to her negative statements and triggers physical stress responses, making her fear a reality. Over time, this becomes a cycle of fear and physical symptoms.

John constantly tells himself, "I'm overweight and unattractive. I have no self-control when it comes to food."

Whenever John feels stressed or receives a negative comment about his appearance, he turns to comfort food. This emotional eating leads to weight gain, reinforcing his negative self-image and beliefs about his lack of self-control.

John's negative self-talk about his body and eating habits creates a mental framework where food becomes both a comfort and a source of guilt. His mind listens to his self-criticism and perpetuates the behavior that aligns with his negative beliefs, creating a vicious cycle of emotional eating and body dissatisfaction.

Lisa often tells herself, "I'm not smart enough to get promoted. I'll never be able to compete with my colleagues." When opportunities for advancement arise, Lisa hesitates to apply or doesn't put in her best effort because she doubts her abilities. This hesitation leads to missed opportunities and reinforces her belief that she isn't capable of progressing in her career.

Lisa's self-doubt and negative self-talk undermine her confidence and performance. Her mind accepts her statements as truth, causing her to act in ways that *confirm her negative beliefs and prevent her from reaching her full potential.*

Michael tells himself, "I can't trust anyone; people always let me down." In his relationships, Michael is constantly suspicious and guarded. He often misinterprets neutral actions as signs of betrayal or disloyalty, leading to conflicts and strained relationships.

Michael's negative self-talk about trust creates a self-fulfilling prophecy. His mind listens to his assertions and reacts by being overly cautious and defensive, which pushes people away and perpetuates his belief that he cannot trust others.

These examples show how this principle ("Your Mind Always Listens and Responds to What You Tell Yourself") operates in everyday life, leading to self-reinforcing patterns that can be difficult to break without positive intervention and change in internal dialogue.

Awareness Is the First Step Toward Change

The subconscious *always* wins—it's trying its best to protect you in the best way it knows how. Your defense mechanisms are ultra-intelligent and adaptive. Your brain does whatever it thinks is necessary to keep you feeling safe, secure, loved, or included even when the results can be disastrous.

Fortunately, it's also changeable. Once we know the underlying trigger, fear, trauma, or baseline belief, we can work way more effectively to change or heal the deep hurt or critical messaging. In fact, change is *only* possible once you've identified and honored your existing patterns. We first have to recognize what the existing pattern is doing for you, and then discover a different way for you to get that thing so that you can stop automatically triggering that safety response.

YOUR TURN: BUILDING AWARENESS AND TRANSFORMING PATTERNS

Find a quiet space where you feel safe and supported. Sit comfortably in a chair or on the floor, allowing your body to relax. Close your eyes if it feels comfortable to do so. Begin by taking a few long, slow breaths in through your nose and out through your mouth. As you breathe, let go of any effort or tension, allowing your breath to become effortless and nourishing.

Imagine a recent event that caused you stress. Visualize it in detail, as if you are watching a scene unfold on a television screen. Notice where you feel tension or discomfort in your body. Breathe into these areas, acknowledging the sensations without judgment. Let yourself fully experience this moment, knowing that every thought or idea causes a physical reaction.

Now, ask yourself, "Does this feeling remind me of a similar experience from my past?" Allow any memories to surface, gently observing them. Notice how your mind moves toward the familiar and away from the unfamiliar. Understand that your current reactions may be deeply connected to past experiences.

Think about the thoughts you had during the stressful event. What did you tell yourself? Identify any negative self-talk or beliefs and keep these specific phrases in your mind or write them down in a journal. Remember, your mind always listens and responds to what you tell yourself. This internal dialogue shapes your reality and influences your mental and physical states.

For each negative statement, imagine an alternative positive affirmation. If you thought, "I'm going to mess up," replace it with, "I am capable and prepared." Visualize yourself saying these positive affirmations with confidence and belief. Feel the shift in your energy as you replace negative thoughts with empowering ones. This is how you align your beliefs with your desired behaviors, acknowledging that opposing ideas cannot be held simultaneously.

GO DEEPER REFLECTION QUESTIONS

- What are the most common negative statements you tell yourself? How do these statements make you feel?
- Can you identify where these negative thoughts might have originated? Do they remind you of messages you received in childhood or from significant people in your life?
- How do these negative self-talk patterns influence your actions and decisions? Can you see specific examples in your life?
- What similarities do you notice between the recent event and past experiences? How do these patterns show up in your current life?
- How can understanding these connections help you change your responses and behaviors in the present?

Allow these reflections to deepen your awareness. Notice how recognizing patterns helps you understand the persistent nature of subconscious beliefs and how identifying the origin of thoughts connects past experiences with current behavior. By challenging your negative self-talk and embracing positive affirmations, you begin to align your actions with your new, empowering beliefs.

Take your time with this exercise. Let the awareness of these principles guide you toward lasting change. Remember, the mind's natural tendency is to maintain the status quo, but with conscious effort and positive reinforcement, you can transform your internal dialogue and create a more fulfilling life.

GO DEEPER AFFIRMATIONS

- I am worthy of love, success, and happiness.
- I am lovable.
- I am enough as I am.
- I acknowledge my past experiences and release their hold on my present.
- I choose new, positive ways to respond to challenges and embrace change.

Now that we've uncovered how the Principles of the Mind can keep us stuck in behaviors we don't want, let's take a pause and allow some hope to enter in. You're not doomed to the life your subconscious mind deems safe and secure. In the next section, we'll uncover how you can begin transforming the baseline beliefs and unhealed hurts that have held you back.

I can't wait.

Chapter 5

Your Past Doesn't Have to Determine Your Future

Kids are awesome, aren't they? As a former kindergarten and preschool teacher, I got the chance to view all sorts of kiddos up close, plus I studied early developmental milestones as part of my education. With the work I do now with adults, I know those developmental milestones don't stop mattering when we grow up. We form and firm up our worldview from birth—whether it's a sunny, positive outlook or a minefield of negativity and shame. When you know how you developed your inner beliefs, it's much easier to begin shifting the ones that no longer serve and protect you the way you'd like.

Right now, take a moment to look back for a moment at little you. What do you love about them? What was something cool about little you? Something that was brilliant before you ever received a judgment, a stern word from a parent, a scolding from a teacher, or bullying from another kid?

Did you love to dance? To sing? To draw or paint? To make things? To sell ice-cold lemonade on the street corner in July? What were you good at? What lit you up?

Everything cool about little you still exists, in some form. That is your unsullied essence; that piece of you existed as pure love and joy before anyone else had anything to say about it.

Your essence, your little you, is the place we're seeking in the hypnosis process. To get there, we have to wade through everything that came after that to make you believe that you were:

- Less than
- Uncool
- Lazy
- Incompetent
- Too loud
- Nerdy
- Bad or wrong
- Weak
- Pushy
- Too big or small
- Not [smart, good, tall, skinny, talented, accomplished, etc.] enough
- Too much
- Different
- Unlovable
- Broken

And that's just a hint of what we pick up about ourselves during childhood and beyond. So why is it so hard to release these critical messages and get on with our successful lives, for crying out loud?

Let's answer that question with a brief and simple dive into the workings of our developing little-kid brains. Because even if we feel like we had a "normal" or "good" childhood from the outside looking in, there's a lot of internal messaging and interpretation about our upbringing that sets up for future behavior bugaboos. Remember, humans are meaning makers.

I hope you'll read this next section with a caring arm around your inner Little One. It's likely they need a ton of understanding and tenderness as you begin picking apart the messages you got as a kid that still hold you back today. And because they are a version of you, you can discover what their unmet needs are and then try to gently meet those needs now in ways that feel expansive and pleasurable—hooray for that! Here we go.

Our thinking, or cognitive, brain doesn't fully come online until we're about twenty-five. Wow! So it's no wonder you look at a teenager and think, "They don't know anything!" It's because they sort of . . . don't.

Even into our early twenties, our impulses govern a ton of what we do; we cannot think all that far into the future. Our executive functioning, which happens in the prefrontal cortex, the part of our brain that lets us organize tasks and plan ahead, is still under construction.

And even much earlier than that, we act and feel our way through life without much logical thought—because our brains simply haven't grown up enough yet. Our early functioning comes largely through our subconscious. So it follows that, as children, we do not have a logical filter—we make sense of what we experience by feeling it and telling stories about it as best we can. Our personal story is almost never an accurate interpretation of the true facts we receive or situations we encounter, yet we believe it to be true.

Let me give an example of how this works: Let's say that little Jane's mom yells at her for spilling a glass of milk. This is something parents do almost automatically, especially if they fear that their child will get hurt stepping on shattered glass, or simply out of exhausted exasperation. Who hasn't been there? Because she got yelled at, Jane thinks she has done a bad thing.

Jane can shake this off fairly easily if it's a onetime event. Let's say her mom repairs the relationship quickly after she yells by apologizing, explaining why she was mad or scared, and then hugging it out. In this case, the glass-shattering incident will be quickly forgotten without becoming a big part of Jane's story. But if it happens regularly and there is no repair, Jane may start to believe that she is bad. She may believe that she's a klutz who can't ever get anything right. She starts to see the world through the lens of the belief that she is someone who cannot be trusted around fragile things. The belief will sink into her subconscious even deeper if her parents continue to reinforce this messaging by using these same words and angry or fearful tones without any explanation.

The messaging takes hold insidiously and begins to color her whole childhood experience. Jane may become shy and fearful of trying new things. Or she may torture herself with anxiety and fear if she does break something else unintentionally. The message of "I shouldn't do that / try that / go there because I'll just break something" may permeate everything she does as she grows up. Her mind will remember most vividly the childhood experiences that prove this belief is true. In all likelihood, Jane drank her milk ninety-nine times without incident for every one time she dropped the glass—but that one time becomes part of her internal story, while the other ninety-nine times are dismissed or forgotten.

So as an adult, Jane feels incompetent most of the time. Her life shrinks painfully to where she cannot give herself permission to do anything she views with desire or excitement. She tells herself that something will always go wrong and she cannot trust herself.

Sure, I'm getting a little dramatic here. But long-term consequences of our early messaging are very real. And I have seen them get even more limiting, more painful, more severe than in the example about Jane. Even when our brains mature and we can use our logic, our inner childhood feelings and stories *always* trump the logic. Here's why.

Developmental Milestones

From birth to adulthood, our brains undergo eight developmental psychosocial milestones. Each stage presents a central conflict that individuals must resolve to develop a healthy personality and acquire basic virtues. Each time we enter one of these stages of maturation, we can experience either a positive or negative outcome. If we achieve the positive outcome, we attain a certain intrinsic attribute. But if we get stuck with the negative outcome, we miss that attribute and are left with its opposite, which is often a detriment to us as we grow up. Each stage builds on the previous ones, emphasizing the importance of successfully navigating each conflict to foster a healthy psychological development.

Dr. Erik Erikson, a renowned psychologist from the late 1950s and '60s, outlined how these eight milestones come about. Everyone has to go through these milestones. Sorry, there's no bypassing them.

If you came through any one of them in a harrowing way with negative aftereffects, that one glitch will influence how you go through all the following steps. I know, total bummer, right? But the good news is, once you recognize a gap in the sequence and any limiting beliefs associated with this gap, with the help of hypnotherapy you can go back and change the outcome.

Before we start investigating your journey through the milestones, bear in mind that psychosocial gaps don't make you a bad person. There's no judgment here. This list is not just one more thing you have to live up to in order to feel okay.

It turns out, no adult sails perfectly through all these milestones—*everyone has gaps*.

This process is just a road map of sorts to let you know where you may have a roadblock in this psychosocial developmental pathway. Once you know where you had some issues, you can address them and still complete this part of your evolution so that your relationships, career, and overall life experience can improve and expand.

Read through this list and see if there are any "light bulb moments" for you about which milestones correspond to gaps. Giving yourself permission to look back at the age ranges may stir the subconscious pot for you and bring up some potentially hard memories. If you find you're feeling distressed, take this section slowly. Be sure to reach out for help and support from your care team, a trusted friend, or someone else who can hold space for your continued exploration at a pace that works for you.

The gaps are not your fault, nor are they necessarily your parents' fault. Most parents do the best they can with the tools and information they have at the time. Read about each milestone and think about your own experience of it, then release any judgment of that experience. You are okay, you are not defective, you are not broken. You also have limitless power to change your experience from here forward—and to do so in a way that feels gentle, supportive, and relaxed.

Stage 1: Trust vs. Mistrust, Birth to Eighteen Months Old

Babies are entirely dependent on their caregivers during this stage. If when they cry, their caregivers consistently bring them the care they need—food, diaper changes, cuddling and contact, sleep, or comfort—they will develop a sense of trust in the world around them. With that trust they can start to form other relationships and feel "okay" even if their sense of security isn't always 100 percent. This success leads to the virtue of hope.

If, on the other hand, the caregiving is inconsistent, inadequate, or nonexistent, their sense of trust will not develop. This mistrust can lead to lasting feelings of suspicion and anxiety, making it difficult for the individual to form secure relationships later in life.

Stage 2: Autonomy vs. Shame, Eighteen Months to Three Years Old

In this stage, kids stay busy working on their independence and developing skills like walking, talking, finer motor functions, balance, and so much more. They need their caregivers to provide reasonable limits to keep them safe while also giving them space to explore and practice what they learn.

Caregivers need to provide the right balance of encouragement and limits to help the child find their voice. Usually a child's first form of self-expression is a strong "No!" The child will also start trying challenging activities—like climbing up and down the stairs, getting dressed each day, reaching to higher shelves, playing in the dirt, making messes, tasting new foods, or lunging for the family cat. Parents can often let these actions' natural consequences guide, shape, and mold the child.

All parents will err on the side of being either too protective, too critical, or too permissive from time to time. As long as the parent recognizes when this happens and course-corrects periodically, the child can still move ahead with a strong sense of self, autonomy, and independence. The child moves on from trusting the world to trusting and healthfully controlling themself. During this stage the child develops the attribute of will.

When the care-giving balance is chronically out of whack, on the other hand, the child grows up without acquiring a sense of will and may have low self-esteem or self-trust, which can show up as intense shame and self-doubt later in life.

Stage 3: Initiative vs. Guilt, Three to Five Years Old

Kids at this age ask relentless questions. They play 100 percent of the time and start discovering how to make friends and get along, or not. They begin learning about leadership and initiative. They may start to suggest, "Let's play pretend right now, and then let's play hide-and-seek!" They learn how to take turns, and how to care about and have fun with their little buddies. A little guilt is a healthy thing too, as children do need to learn what happens when they overstep a boundary, say a hurtful thing, or do something that harms someone else.

When parents encourage their child's exploration, honor their questions, even when they are beyond annoying, and set up opportunities for free and natural play with other kids in a variety of environments, their child acquires initiative and purpose.

When parents continually brush off their child or treat them as a nuisance, the child feels guilty and ashamed. This can translate into a feeling of being "too much" as an adult, so they stay small, self-deprecating, diminutive, or "seen and not heard."

Stage 4: Industry vs. Inferiority, Five to Twelve Years Old

In these crucial learning years, children want to gain approval for the tasks they accomplish that society deems valuable, like reading, writing, and math in school. Peer groups assume new importance as kids learn to interact more meaningfully within their friend circles and gain more social acceptance, or not. Kids strive for ever-increasing independence and begin to focus internally on justice, fairness, or belonging over pleasing their caregivers.

When children at this age receive encouragement for their continued exploration and learning valuable skills, they become confident and feel proud of all they can do. This leads them to internalize the attribute of competence.

When kids struggle to achieve, get overly criticized or cut down for "failure," or feel stifled and restricted in their independence, they can doubt their abilities or potential and feel inferior.

While too much failure or criticism can cause a gap in this stage, some struggle during this stage is good. When a child tries and fails a few times at a skill, they learn to balance their pride with modesty.

Stage 5: Identity vs. Role Confusion, Twelve to Eighteen Years Old

Independence grows as children start looking toward the future at what they'd like to be and do—how they may want to live their lives as adults. At this stage, a child may consider things like what college to attend, what jobs seem exciting or inviting, places they want to explore, goals for new or existing activities, or whether they want to get married and raise a family someday. "Finding themselves" (that is, exploring several identity markers) is paramount to this age and stage of development.

Parents who observe, encourage, and listen to their teens about these key identity pieces may foster the attribute of fidelity, and the teen will learn how to like, care about, and get along with others even when they don't agree or share the same roles, or when they have different identity lenses. Teens with fidelity are often comfortable with their "role" in society and the way they fit into the world around them.

When teens are forced into a certain role—like when they hear statements such as "you *will* go to college" "gay relationships are sinful and bad," or "women shouldn't be scientists"—they can leave adolescence without a clear sense of who they are and how they fit into our current culture. This confusion is sometimes called an *identity crisis* and can have far-reaching impacts into adulthood.

Stage 6: Intimacy vs. Isolation, Eighteen to Forty Years Old

In this lengthy stage, we develop our comfort and skill with relational intimacy. We can enter into marriage, partnership, and other iterations of close relationships that allow us to see others clearly and be seen at deeper levels in turn.

Completing this stage successfully might mean that we find comfort and security in marriage or long-term partnership, become a parent, or have several key friendships that sustain and fulfill us. We learn how to deeply care for ourselves and others in this stage, and what that care looks like in a practical, actionable sense. The attribute we can attain at this stage is love.

The negative inverse of this attribute is fear of intimacy or commitment, which may bring about depression, anxiety, and even physical health problems stemming from isolation.

Stage 7: Generativity vs. Stagnation, Forty to Sixty-Five Years Old

Here is where we seek and discover our ability to create or nurture something that will outlast us. Examples include raising children, launching a professional mentorship of someone younger than you at work, developing an innovative new idea that stands the test of time, inventing a tangible object that betters the lives of many, writing and publishing a book, and getting involved in your community or a cause about which you care deeply.

When we accomplish what we hoped for our lives in this stage, we feel useful, timeless, successful, and relevant. Successful navigation of this stage gives us the gift of care.

If we fail during this stage, our community connection and significance can feel shallow and fleeting. At this end are stagnation and nonproductivenss, which can make us feel depressed, invisible, and like our lives didn't really mean much in the grand scheme of humanity.

Stage 8: Ego Integrity vs. Despair, Sixty-Five Years Old Till Death

This powerful stage is where we typically look back on our lives with a critical eye. Did we accomplish what we set out to do in our lives? What major mistakes did we make along the way? What triumphs and successes lit the way forward? What are our major regrets? Will anyone care about our contributions?

If we come up feeling even a little satisfied that we did our best, that who and what we are matters, and that we didn't leave a crucial stone unturned or a critical experience undone, we receive the gift of Ego Integrity.

But even despair is still a gift in this stage, because it's the *balance* of the two that makes for a full life. Of course we will remember with despair those moments where we didn't exactly shine in our humanity. But when you can even out the score by seeing the good and the bad together, you receive the gift of wisdom—an acknowledgment of the imperfect completeness of your life, without fear of accepting the truth of the hard times or mistakes you made along the way.

People who see their lives as meaningless, unproductive, or riddled with guilt tend to despair in greater measure, which can also bring about depression and shame at this late life stage.

You Are Not Broken!

Whew! Take a deep breath. Even if you uncovered several psychosocial milestones you may lack in their fullest measure, you're still okay. Because guess what? No one travels this developmental pathway perfectly. And if we did, we wouldn't be imperfectly human, and life would sure be . . . boring.

Adversity and developmental gaps can be the fuel that stokes us to reach for something better in our lives, without relentless pressure or striving. Recovery and change can take a long time, but changes do happen in so many surprising ways with practice and support.

The hardest part of change is actually seeing the gaps. Once you acknowledge what you lack and what you'd like to have, you can go about the business of getting it, in ways that calm your nervous system and reinforce your deepest desires for yourself. Remember, only you can decide what it looks like to pass a particular milestone; it doesn't matter what someone else thinks you should want.

> **YOUR TURN: EXPLORE YOUR DEVELOPMENTAL ATTRIBUTES**
>
> Look back at each of these eight stages. Focus primarily on stages one through five, as those are your childhood years. Allow some memories to come up for you from each stage. Keep a lens of curiosity, not judgment, as you remember how or when you achieved some of the attributes listed above, or where the obvious gaps are for you.
>
> Remember to have a ton of compassion for yourself as you look back on your upbringing. Keep in mind that your resources and understanding were limited as a child and your executive functioning wasn't fully developed. Give yourself some grace for the choices you made in your past.
>
> We will continue to learn how to understand and forgive all the younger versions of yourself in the upcoming chapters. If this process of remembering feels big or overwhelming, know that you can stop at any time and seek the professional or friendly support you need. In the next chapter, I'll outline how to make this healing process manageable and gentle as you move forward.

Chapter 6

Introduction to Parts Work and Internal Family Systems in Hypnotherapy

Do you ever feel like different parts of you are pulling in opposite directions? Maybe there's a part of you that wants to take a bold step forward in your career, but another part holds you back with fears and doubts. Or perhaps you've found yourself repeatedly engaging in behaviors that you know aren't good for you, but you can't seem to stop. These internal conflicts are a common human experience and can be deeply perplexing and frustrating.

In hypnotherapy, this phenomenon is understood through the concept of "Parts Work." Imagine your mind as a community made up of various members, each with its own voice, desires, and roles. Some of these members may be Protectors, working tirelessly to keep you safe based on past experiences. Others might be younger versions of you that have been tucked away in your memory, carrying the wounds and burdens that you've accumulated over your lifetime. These parts, each with their unique perspectives, can sometimes be at odds with one another, leading to the internal struggles you experience.

Parts Work is a powerful therapeutic approach that helps you identify, understand, and harmonize these different aspects of yourself. By acknowledging and communicating with these parts, you can begin to resolve internal conflicts, heal past traumas, and integrate these diverse elements into a cohesive and harmonious whole. This process can lead to profound personal growth, increased self-awareness, and greater emotional balance.

The foundations of Parts Work in hypnotherapy were significantly influenced by Charles Tebbetts, who developed parts therapy to address these internal divisions. His innovative methods have led the way in the field, but Tebbetts was not alone. Other pioneers like Milton Erickson, John G. Watkins, and Richard Schwartz have also made substantial contributions, each adding their unique insights and techniques to the practice of Parts Work.

Milton Erickson's use of storytelling and metaphors, John G. Watkins's Ego-State Therapy, and, more recently, Richard Schwartz's Internal Family Systems (IFS) model have all enriched the understanding and application of Parts Work. These approaches highlight the importance of recognizing that each part, no matter how disruptive it may seem, has a positive intention and a role in your overall well-being.

In this chapter, we'll explore the essential concepts of Parts Work, delving into the techniques and philosophies that underpin this transformative approach. We'll look at how understanding the multiplicity of the mind and fostering communication between parts can lead to significant breakthroughs in personal evolution. By the end of this chapter, you'll have a deeper appreciation for the complexity of your inner world and the tools to begin navigating it more effectively.

Important Concepts of Parts Work

The mind is not a singular entity but is composed of various parts, each with its own thoughts, feelings, and behaviors. We'll discuss parts like your inner child and your Protector Parts as we move through the rest of this narrative together. These pieces of the Whole You reside in every human. In Parts Work used in hypnotherapy, the hypnotherapist helps the client identify and communicate with these different parts. The goal is to understand the roles and purposes of each part, address conflicts, and integrate the parts into a harmonious whole.

Each part has its own perspective and emotions, and the goal is to integrate these parts harmoniously. Each of our parts has feelings and sensations. They carry burdens and enjoy triumphs. It's like you actually have several functioning people within you all at the same time. For example, there's likely a manager-like part of you that feels very organized and on top of things, and appears responsible most of the time.

There may also be a part of you that's a couch potato and never has much motivation to do anything other than open a bag of chips and zone out in front of the TV. That part of you might have taken on the sluggish role to counteract the Responsible Part so that you don't burn out completely and you can get some rest and recovery once in a while.

It's important to remember that both of these parts, and all the rest of your parts, have a positive intent in your life, even if it doesn't look that way from the outside. They're *all* trying to keep you safe and have your needs met in the only ways they know how.

Your Responsible Part may have taken on this role as a kid to get validation and love from your mom, dad, or caregiver.

Responsible You is characterized as a *Proactive Part*, while Couch Potato You is known as a *Reactive Part*. Both of these parts can be known as *Protector Parts*.

Your Proactive Parts are born out of a need for love, acceptance, belonging, or visibility. Your Reactive Parts develop as a way to relieve pain (emotional and physical), and balance the Proactive Parts that would run amok otherwise. They both believe they're helping you in the best way they can.

In Parts Work, a distinction is made between the core or True Self and the various parts. The Self is the central, undamaged essence of a person, capable of leading the internal system. Richard Schwartz highlights the importance of the Self as a compassionate and confident leader of the internal family.

Internal Conflict and Resolution

Understanding that internal conflicts often arise when different parts have opposing needs or desires is crucial. These conflicts can cause significant psychological distress and may manifest as indecision, anxiety, or self-sabotaging behaviors. Parts therapy aims to mediate these conflicts, fostering dialogue and understanding between the conflicting parts, which can lead to resolution and internal harmony.

Non-Pathologizing Approach

A key tenet of Parts Work is the non-pathologizing approach to each part of the self. This means recognizing that all parts, even those exhibiting maladaptive behaviors, have positive intentions. They are often protective mechanisms developed in response to past experiences. By understanding and appreciating the roles these parts play, clients can work toward integrating them rather than viewing them as problematic or pathological.

Hypnotic Techniques and Accessing the Subconscious

Hypnosis is often used to facilitate Parts Work because it allows for direct communication with the subconscious mind, where these parts reside. Through hypnosis, clients can access and engage with their parts more effectively, uncovering hidden memories and motivations that drive their behaviors. This process can lead to deeper insights and more profound healing.

By exploring and understanding these concepts, you can begin to recognize the positive intentions behind even the most challenging parts of yourself. Through Parts Work, you will learn to harmonize these aspects, leading to a more integrated and balanced sense of self. This chapter aims to provide you with the knowledge and tools to embark on this journey of self-discovery and healing. For more information on the evolution of Parts Work and Dr. Schwartz's work and publications, refer to the resources at the end of this book.

PROACTIVE AND REACTIVE PARTS IN ACTION

As you read through the following examples of proactive and reactive protective parts, consider how your own parts show up in your life presently and how they may have developed.

Proactive Parts

Lisa's mom was diagnosed with breast cancer when she was five. She went through chemo and radiation multiple times and was ill for about five years. She passed away when Lisa was ten. From the original diagnosis and through all of the treatments, Lisa learned she needed to be a good girl and take care of her mom. She learned there was no room for her needs. She believed her needs didn't matter.

This "good girl" part always followed the rules and became a People Pleaser to protect her from her mom leaving and abandoning her. Even when Lisa was an adult, the protective part worked extremely hard to make sure the people she loved didn't leave her. She continued to be a "good girl" and a People Pleaser to feel safe.

Reactive Parts

When Kylee was eight, she was in a car accident with her mom and younger sister. Her mom was badly injured and her younger sister died in the accident. Kylee survived and had only minor injuries. After this incident, her mom was severely depressed and continued to be in pain all the time. The survivor's guilt and witnessing her mom's sadness was so painful for Kylee that she began to use food to soothe and numb her emotional pain and guilt. All Kylee knew was that food made her feel better for a short time at least. Kylee felt like she didn't deserve to live when her sister died and her mom was in so much pain, so she just ate until she didn't feel the pain. This reactive behavior continued into her adult years whenever she felt scared, anxious, sad, ashamed, or unworthy.

YOUR TURN:
LET YOUR PARTS INTRODUCE THEMSELVES

Here's a gentle activity you can use to start discovering and understanding some of your Protector Parts that want to keep you safe and secure, even if they go about it in ways that no longer serve you, and how to start powerfully shifting them to make changes in your life.

Begin by finding a comfortable space where you can sit or lie down without interruptions. Allow yourself to get into a meditative state, perhaps starting with a few deep breaths or playing some calming music to help set the mood. As you relax, connect with your True Self, embracing the qualities of compassion, caring, and curiosity. Let these qualities fill your awareness, creating a sense of calm and openness.

With your eyes closed or gaze looking softly down, look inward and identify a part of you that feels like it's stopping or blocking you from living the life you desire. This part might sound critical, anxious, or "perfect," and could remind you of your mom, dad, sibling, or another source of negativity from your childhood. As you focus on this part, notice any sensations, colors, textures, or images that arise. How old is this part? What does it sound like? What does it look like? How is it feeling right now? Take your time to fully observe and connect with these characteristics.

Ask this part, "What is your role?" or "What is your purpose?" Listen with curiosity and compassion, allowing the response to come through without judgment. Get to know this part in as much detail as possible, understanding its fears for you, what it believes would happen if it stopped doing its job, and its needs. Witness this part fully and feel gratitude for how it has been serving you up to this point in your life. Take as long as you need with this process and allow it to unfold organically without judgment.

When you feel the process is complete, thank the part for showing up and sharing with you, acknowledging its efforts to help you in its own way. Take a few breaths and gradually come back to full awareness.

GO DEEPER REFLECTION QUESTIONS

Spend a few moments writing what you experienced in your journal. You can use the following questions to help guide you if needed:

- What did you learn about this part of yourself?
- How has it been serving you?
- How does this part affect your emotions and behaviors in your daily life? Are there particular situations where it becomes more prominent?
- How can you meet those needs in another way that aligns with the person you are today?

GO DEEPER AFFIRMATIONS

- I accept all parts of myself with compassion and understanding.
- I embrace the harmony and balance within my inner world.
- I am grateful for the protection and guidance my inner parts have provided me.

The only way to create change in your life is to become fully aware of what's going on inside you in the present. Your parts are part of that "now" landscape. After you uncover them, you'll also need to accept them—and the help they've offered to you up to this point.

Remember that your parts are created to keep you safe, moving toward "pleasure" (even if it's a warped definition of what is pleasurable), and in the familiar. If you do not take the time to discover, dissect, and replace them, you'll inevitably keep repeating the same behaviors that got you where you are now.

And it's okay. Always remember that you're not broken—your mind is chugging along in exactly the way it was designed to do. But now that you have some more insight into your Protector Parts, the pathway to real and lasting change can reveal itself to you.

One of the first real action steps in hypnotherapy is to heal little you inside you who adopted those limiting beliefs in the first place, to stay safe, sane, and protected. Let's let little you have some of your much-needed attention, shall we?

Chapter 7

Who Are Your Protectors Guarding? (Hint: Your Inner Child)

Inner child work can be hard and you'll be invited to feel sometimes-intense emotions. Many clients wonder why they have to go back into the past, because it can be painful, triggering, and depressing, and there's nothing you can do about what's already happened. But I'm here to tell you that the meaning you make of the past is more changeable than you think. You can begin to change your relationship with your past experiences.

Here's why healing your inner child is crucial to changing your behaviors, beliefs, and entire life:

If your inner child has emotional wounds and safety gaps (remember all those milestones from Chapter 5?), they will continue to run the show from the wounded place inside of you. The little you (and your Protectors) will always be in the driver's seat until you meet the core needs you missed and heal the wounds from your past.

The reason your inner child and the Protector Parts of you are "loud" is that they desperately want a different outcome than the one that wounded you in the first place. Our minds continue to reexperience the painful situations we endured so that we have a chance to edit the past and end up with a different future. It's like we need an opportunity for a do-over.

It's no surprise that you keep choosing the same problematic partners, the same tiresome jobs and bosses, and the same sticky situations that invite you to come to your inner child's aid as a grown-up. You'll keep coming back to the same circumstances until you can finally learn the lesson that's hidden for you there. In other words, you'll need to give yourself whatever you didn't receive from your parents or caregivers, before any meaningful change can occur.

Imagine for a moment that your inner child exists as a real being. They're angry, sad, and scared because of trauma (big or small) or abandonment (acute or chronic). They generally don't believe that the world is safe, kind, or generous. What do angry, sad, and scared little kids do when their feelings are so big? They yell, break things, bang on furniture, and otherwise create chaos trying to get their (very valid) needs met. Or they shut down, shut the people who love them out, and bottle everything up so no one can see how much they're hurting. Their feelings also easily overwhelm their little bodies, so they construct protective coping behaviors (or "parts") to shield themselves from the emotional overwhelm of the pain they must endure.

Your Protector Parts come online at first in childhood to protect the most vulnerable parts of yourself. When your inner child is so wounded and vulnerable, your parts must take on the extreme protective roles to shield you from pain.

Here's the bad news. The parts of you that protect your inner child get louder and more insistent as time goes on—whenever that inner child feels triggered or threatened. When a situation in your present-day life reminds you of your childhood wounds subconsciously, your wounded inner child reactivates, sending your Protector Parts into overdrive.

As years go by, your protective parts, like your inner critic or Perfectionist, get even more dominant so that your inner child doesn't have to feel overwhelming feelings. But those Protectors also can wreak havoc on your physical health, with such issues as tension headaches, inflammation, heart attacks, and gut problems. The Protectors can also impact your mental well-being in the form of anxiety, depression, or PTSD symptoms. Your Protectors can even prevent you from having meaningful, safe, and rewarding relationships, or enjoying a sense of safety and joy in your own body.

Your Protectors cause trouble. For example they might force you to be "perfect" in every way so that you'll gain approval and safety, even if it means you have chronic heartburn and off-the-charts anxiety. Or they might destroy all your relationships because real intimacy and vulnerability make you want to crawl out of your skin.

Fun fact: Your Protectors will always respond to your environment exactly as they did when you were three, five, eight, or fourteen years old. They believe that you're a little kid who needs their help, even though you're an adult. For example, if your mother becomes hypercritical of your academic performance when you enter high school, you may develop a fierce inner critic. The inner critic believes it is protecting you by motivating you to work harder, therefore preventing criticism from outer sources. The inner critic will continue to respond to your life events as if you are still a young teenager, even as you move into adulthood.

As we begin this inner child healing work, know that it can be a challenge to look back. It's also important to keep in mind that this process is not about reliving every detail of your painful past; that's not necessary to heal and it is not actually possible to relive the past. It *is* crucial to review your past at a level that allows your inner child to be heard and for their needs to be met today by you. Your inner child must obtain those early milestones of safety, security, and trust that they somehow missed out on along the way.

There are specific details of the past that have caused you to form harmful beliefs about yourself and subconscious behavior patterns you don't love and can't stop. When you look back consciously and carefully, you can change your relationship to those memories and your responses.

Important Notes to Remember

You cannot change the events of the past, but you *can* change your relationship and response to them! You can change your interpretation, or the meaning you make, of your past.

Here's some good news: You are the perfect person to help your inner child, because you were that Little One. You have a front-row seat to the original experience, and you are an expert on you.

I also highly recommend getting outside support while you do your inner child healing. This support could be a trusted friend who can listen without judging or trying to fix you. It could be a supportive community like a sharing circle or twelve-step program. This support is also what I offer during my private hypnotherapy sessions. We look back on your life together as gently as possible at the pace that works for you. We uncover one developmental gap at a time, one limiting belief at a time, and one hurtful past event at a time. When we do this slowly and gently, you can learn, adapt, and take action to feel better more quickly.

Once you understand the issue that is getting in your way and when in your life this issue emerged, you can start to look at your younger self from that stage. What were you feeling then? What was going on in your world? How did you respond to events and circumstances around you? What felt hard, what felt easy, and what support did you have, if any?

When you answer these questions from your "now" vantage point, you can begin to see why parts of you stepped up to "protect" your Little One and how they did that.

This healing is all about witnessing, validating, and re-parenting your inner child by creating safety and meeting their needs. It may take some practice to become the parent of yourself. And that's completely okay. Here's an example of how that practice can evolve with time and intention.

Overcoming Protector Parts in Action

Meet Jonathan. He grew up in a chaotic household where his dad was an alcoholic and his mom was a classic enabler. Jonathan learned very early to walk on eggshells around his dad because he never knew what version of him he was going to get—anything from to a perfectly nice guy to harmful words or even violence.

Jonathan unconsciously developed a Protector Part of a harsh inner critic to keep himself small and invisible, so as not to set off the angry and hurtful version of his father. The self-talk of the inner critic offered hurtful messages before anyone else could. The job of the inner critic was to protect Jonathan, to keep him in line and out of the line of fire of his unpredictable father.

Jonathan's inner critic has stuck around all of his life, keeping him small and invisible, because that part still thinks he is five years old.

When he is able to heal the five-year-old part of himself by helping him feel safe, secure, valued, and trusting, Jonathan's inner critic can begin to relax and step back, because the five-year-old version of him is now being protected by his adult self. When Jonathan takes on the role of Protector, this allows his inner critic to let go of the protective role.

When the inner critic doesn't feel the need to protect the five-year-old anymore, it can choose to take on another job, one that it is better suited for. For example, it might become the Inner Cheerleader, offering confidence, support, and motivation.

Steps for Inner Child Healing

The moments in your present when you feel triggered, or past wounded parts of you are activated, these moments are opportunities for healing. These are glimpses into your past wounding. If you ever find yourself questioning your actions or saying something along the lines of "that's so unlike me," you are likely experiencing a reactivated wounded younger version of you. During these times you may feel as if you are time traveling.

To heal little you, you'll need to go back and figure out what they needed at the time of the original wounding. They probably needed actual physical safety, to be a child, and to be seen, heard, and understood.

You can look at ways to provide these needs for your inner child today. You'll need to continue this work on an ongoing basis because it will take time and consistency for your inner child to feel safe and for your Protector Parts to step back. If you experienced abandonment or rejection in your past, the last thing you want to do is abandon or reject your inner child after first making a connection with them.

Check in with your inner child daily in the beginning of your healing process to make sure they don't feel abandoned or rejected. Bring them along in your imagination to the fun activities you get to do each week, like taking walks or hanging out with your friends. You can also choose to spend time doing the things you loved to do as a child but don't often give yourself the pleasure of doing anymore as an adult.

When was the last time you swung on a playground swing? Or rode on a roller coaster? Or visited the library and let yourself stay and read whatever you wanted? Or even sampled a fun ice cream flavor on a hot summer day?

If you have young children of your own and take them on outings and events, be sure to invite your inner child to come along and enjoy the fun. They can live forever, safely, in your heart and home to begin to feel safer and more secure so that your Protector Parts can continue to stand down.

A word of caution if you have children: Your children's developmental stages can often reactivate your own childhood wounds. When you find yourself triggered by interaction with your children, take some time to ask yourself how the situation reminds you of your past, and how you can comfort and support the wounded child within you.

Also note: If you've tried really hard to parent differently than your parents did, your inner child may become a little jealous of your wonderful parenting. This is a great opportunity to include your inner child as you raise your children up to receive what you didn't when you were their age.

Working with the Inevitable Resistance to Healing Your Inner Child

You may have a Protector Part pop up in resistance when you begin to do this work. That part may sound something like, "This is silly. I can't change the past, so why go back there?" or "inner child healing is woo-woo hogwash, it's way too 'out there' to be effective. No thanks!"

The resistance that you may feel when trying this process, or even considering this process, is likely a protective strategy. If you had a lot of difficult emotions or traumatic experiences when you were young, it will most definitely feel scary to review the past. Your mind doesn't want to feel the painful emotions or overwhelm from that hard time in your life, which is why we develop our protective or reactive parts.

It's natural to be nervous, anxious, or afraid of looking back at the painful or traumatic parts of your life. Remember, it's crucial to have support and to proceed at a pace that lets you review without feeling overwhelmed, but still allows you to feel the feelings and heal the hurts as an adult. The only way out is through, but you can absolutely do it.

When resistance comes up, ask yourself, "How is the resistance serving me?" Just like your inner critic, the resistance is likely a protective part. When you show understanding and appreciation for the protection, this part can step back and allow you to explore more deeply.

In addition, I would suggest working with the sensations you experience in the present moment if looking at the past is still too overwhelming. What I mean by this is to stay present with what you are feeling in the moment, as it happens, and don't worry about looking at your past until you are ready. Seek out the support of a trauma-informed therapist, somatic therapist, or coach to help guide you.

We'll continue to work gently with healing your inner child in the next chapters, too. I'm here with you all the way.

PROTECTORS IN ACTION

Samantha is a thirty-five-year-old woman who sought out hypnotherapy because she was struggling with chronic self-doubt and fear of abandonment. She had a pattern of entering toxic relationships that mirrored her parents' tumultuous marriage. Samantha had just ended yet another long-term relationship, and that was the catalyst for her to make the hypnotherapy appointment with me.

In our session, Samantha uncovered subconscious beliefs about herself and relationships stemming from her childhood experience, including:

- It wasn't safe to be herself.
- She had to please her mom so as not to upset her.
- She was unlovable and unworthy.

Samantha's early years in a difficult household, witnessing frequent arguments and emotional volatility, were compounded by her parents' divorce when she was eight years old. At the end of all that, Samantha was left feeling abandoned and unlovable. Everything Samantha experienced shaped her belief that she was unworthy of love and likely to be abandoned.

In any new relationship that Samantha began as an adult, she felt doomed to fail because her mind kept playing out the familiar in hopes of getting a different outcome. When each relationship inevitably began delivering challenges, which are present in every relationship, healthy or not, Samantha's Protectors sprang into action. Her Protectors, which include People Pleaser and Self-Hiding, sabotaged the relationships.

Samantha could never be fully herself with a partner because her Protectors always told her it wasn't safe.

Samantha's inner messaging told her that she was unlovable and likely to be abandoned, so she kept choosing situations that reinforced this belief. Remember, our mind likes to be "right," which equates to a distorted sense of pleasure. Better to be miserable in the "known" than to be brave in the unknown and undertake an intolerable risk!

Samantha and I worked on healing her inner child. In our sessions, Samantha came to understand that her fear of abandonment and her toxic relationship patterns were connected to her childhood events, not to her as a person. She was able to convince herself that she was inherently good and lovable, two milestones she missed out on as a kid.

Samantha communicated with her inner child through guided imagery, hypnotherapy, and some intentional daily practices after our session. As she connected more dots from her past, she had some profound emotional breakthroughs while witnessing and validating her inner child's pain.

Samantha committed to re-parenting her inner child by providing the love and support she'd never received. Samantha used daily check-ins with her inner child and consistently engaged "Little Samantha" in activities that delivered lots of joy and nurturing.

Samantha invited her inner child to come along with her to spend time in nature, dance, or do art, which was everything she loved doing as a kid! On her follow-up appointment, Samantha shared how doing these new rituals helped her feel less triggered in her present life—so much so that she had begun a new, healthier relationship!

YOUR TURN: CONNECT WITH YOUR YOUNGER SELF FOR HEALING AND LOVE

Try this meditation to gently begin seeing, hearing, and healing the Little One within you. Remember, they're likely desperate to be seen and loved, even if they are also afraid to speak up.

Pro tip: Record yourself reading this exercise out loud. Most smartphones have the capability to voice record. Then play it back for your very own customized meditation experience.

Make yourself comfortable and close your eyes when you are ready. Take three or four cleansing breaths, in through your nose and out through your mouth. Make any shifts or adjustments to your posture or your environment to be as comfortable and safe as possible.

As you allow your physical body to continue softening and relaxing, and your thinking mind to slow down, offer this internal request: "May this experience and healing process be supportive and in alignment with the highest good of all concerned."

With a sense of safety in your body, connect with the support beneath you. Imagine a connecting cord extending from the base of your spine, reaching below the surface beneath you and deep into the earth. Allow yourself to feel connected to the earth's energy and stability.

Next, visualize a bright, radiant light above your head as a protective energy. This light is flowing down into your body, filling you with warmth and love. Welcome both the support of the earth beneath you and this protective energy to be present during this experience.

Now, begin to locate and make a connection with your True Self. This is the truest you that is wise, loving, and compassionate. Your truest self is curious and caring. Imagine your Self to be leading your experience through this exploration. This is helpful to avoid the protective parts trying to be in the driver's seat of your experience.

With earth's energy and connection to your Self, you are safe as I guide you through the process of meeting and healing your inner child. Trust that you are safe, supported, and held in this process.

Imagine a peaceful and safe place in your mind. This can be a real place you've been to before, or a place that exists only in your imagination. Allow yourself to feel relaxed and at ease in this place.

In this safe space in your mind, call to mind a younger version of yourself from an age where you may have needed a little safety and support, a time when you needed love and to know everything was going to be okay. You may see a photo of yourself in your mind or remember an event from your past. Whatever shows up is perfect, and remember you are reviewing the past, not reliving the past.

Let go of the stories and labels that may show up, and simply be with this younger you. If it feels right to you, place one hand on your belly and one on your heart to connect on a deeper level with yourself and your inner child.

Imagine your inner child standing in front of you, looking up at you with wide eyes and a hopeful expression. Take a moment to notice any emotions that may come up, and be with those feelings.

Your inner child recognizes you as their adult self. Begin to build trust with them. Tell your inner child that you are here to take care of them and meet their needs. You are here to protect them if they need it. Ask them if there's anything they need from you at this moment.

Listen to what your inner child has to say and offer reassurance, kindness, and compassion. Let your inner child know that you are here for them and that you love and accept them just as they are.

Acknowledge and validate the feelings of your younger self. It's okay to feel these emotions, and it's important to give yourself permission to feel them fully. Be there with your inner child to support them in any way they need and offer them unconditional love.

Ask your inner child what they need from you in order to feel safe, loved, and nurtured. Listen to what they have to say without judgment or criticism.

Do they need safety and the feeling of being protected, secure, and free from harm? Do they need love and the feeling of being cared for, valued, and appreciated? Do they need nurturance and the feeling of being nourished, supported, and encouraged? Do they need to have the opportunity to be a child, including playfulness, having fun, being creative, and free to express themselves?

Take some time to really hear all they have to say, witness their emotions, and validate their experience.

Invite your inner child to come live in your heart in the present where you can make sure they are safe, loved, and never alone. You are becoming the inner parent of your younger self. As their parent, your job is to meet their needs, take care of them, and love them unconditionally.

Imagine your younger self merging into your heart so you can keep them safe. Your inner child is always in your heart from now on.

Take a deep breath in and feel your heart opening, then as you breathe out, feel the gentle compression as if your lungs are giving your heart, and your inner child, a hug. With this merging, you can relax and heal on an even deeper level.

Tell your younger self that they matter, they are relevant, they are lovable, and they are good enough as they are. Tell them that you will love them unconditionally and keep them safe.

You can say:

- I am here to protect you and keep you safe.
- You don't have to worry about anything.
- I love you just the way you are, and I always will.
- You are precious and valuable to me.
- Tell them anything else you know they need to hear.

Now imagine yourself and your inner child being surrounded by a warm and loving light. This light represents healing and unconditional love. As you focus on this light, imagine it surrounding and enveloping you both, helping to heal any past wounds. Imagine sending healing and love to your younger self, and to the parts of you that are still wounded or hurting.

As you continue to focus on the light, imagine any negative thoughts or beliefs melting away, replaced by positive and empowering ones. Spend a few minutes in this peaceful and healing state, allowing your inner child to feel loved and supported.

Take a moment to reflect on your own journey and how you've come to be the person you are today. Offer yourself kindness, compassion, and understanding.

Now offer gratitude for yourself and your inner child. Thank yourself for taking the time to connect with your inner child and meet their needs. Acknowledge the progress you've made and the love and compassion you've shown yourself.

Take a deep breath and visualize yourself and your inner child feeling happy, safe, and loved. When you're ready, slowly open your eyes and take a few deep breaths.

Remember, healing your inner child is a process that takes time and may involve working with a professional. It's important to be patient with yourself and to practice self-care and self-compassion as you work through these crucial reflections. That means gently noticing when your Protector parts get louder, saying, "This is so stupid, I'm not doing it!" or "This will never work; I'm better off the way I am right now." If you feel called to continue this deeply healing process, consider a personalized hypnotherapy session, or speak with a helping professional you trust.

GO DEEPER REFLECTION QUESTIONS

- What emotions does your inner child experience?
- Identify the Protector Parts that come online to shield your inner child. How do these parts try to protect you, and in what situations do they become most active?

- What present-day situations trigger your inner child's fears or insecurities? How do these triggers relate to past experiences?

- How can you provide the love, safety, and validation your inner child needs today? What daily practices can help you re-parent your inner child?

GO DEEPER AFFIRMATIONS

- I am here to protect and keep my inner child safe. Together, we are secure.

- I love and accept my inner child just as they are. They are precious and valuable.

- All parts of me are welcome and valued.

These reflection questions and affirmations are designed to help you delve deeper into the process of healing your inner child, fostering a sense of safety, love, and understanding. By engaging with these exercises regularly, you can begin to transform your relationship with your past and create a more harmonious and fulfilling present.

Chapter 8

Connect with Your Inner Child

So many of our present-day issues and challenges stem from things that happened when we were kids or even young adults. While you can certainly make plenty of changes in your life without digging up too much of the past, when you encounter a habit or behavior that won't budge no matter what you try, it's likely that issue has deeper roots.

As we set the stage for successful hypnotherapy that results in the life changes you wish to see, it's paramount to look into your early past. Here's why:

- Our past impacts our present in many ways.

- As children, we make meaning out of our experiences, which forms our beliefs about ourselves.

- Because our prefrontal cortex, the logical part of our brain, isn't yet fully formed, these meanings are much more based on instinct and emotion than logic or fact.

- Our minds are meaning makers. It's impossible to experience anything without assigning a story to it—and most often, that story will be one you first created at an early age.

- Our experiences and beliefs make up our inner world, the lens through which we see our outer world.

Understanding How Our Paradigms Shape Our Perception

Imagine a very adorable, lovable cross-eyed rhino painting several lovely scenes outdoors. As you observe her artwork, you'll notice that every scene she paints contains a prominent horn. This isn't because she's fixated on horns, but because it's the image right in front of her face, dominating her field of vision. She cannot see anything that doesn't have the horn in the view; it's her only perspective and shapes the way she interprets her surroundings.

This charming rhino artist perfectly illustrates how our own experiences and paradigms shape our view of the world. Just like the rhino, we each have a "horn"—a particular set of experiences, beliefs, and biases—that influences how we see and interpret everything around us. This is the lens through which we view our reality, often without even realizing it.

From a young age, our experiences start to form these lenses. The way our parents treated us, the messages we received from society, our successes and failures, and the emotional and physical environments we were exposed to all contribute to the "horn" in our perspective. Over time, these experiences solidify into a set of paradigms that influence how we see ourselves and the world.

For instance, if you grew up in a household where you were constantly criticized, your "horn" might be a deep-seated belief that you're not good enough. Consequently, you might interpret neutral feedback at work as harsh criticism, or see a partner's constructive comment as a personal attack. This happens not because the feedback or comment is inherently negative, but because your paradigm filters it through the lens of your past experiences.

Just like the rhino can't see beyond her horn without changing her perspective, we often can't see beyond our ingrained beliefs and experiences. The process of inner work, such as parts therapy and inner child healing, helps us to recognize our "horns" and learn to see the world from a broader, more objective perspective. By understanding and healing the parts of us that formed these paradigms, we can start to perceive life more clearly and respond to it in healthier, more adaptive ways.

This understanding is crucial for personal growth. By becoming aware of the lenses through which we view the world, we can begin to challenge and change them. This transformation allows us to interact with our environment in ways that are more aligned with our true selves, rather than being dictated by past wounds and outdated beliefs.

Plus, if there is *trauma* in your background, your brain machinery gets hijacked even further as you try to cope as best you can with the painful or harmful thing that happened to you. Traumatic events color the way we interpret our experiences and, like the rhino, we cannot see a world where we don't know the trauma.

If you've never been shown anything else besides your own horn, it takes something from outside yourself to give you another view of what's possible.

In the "Your Turn" section at the end of this chapter, there is an exercise in cracking the door on your past—and bringing in some new perspective for you—so you can *stop* seeing just the horn, and start seeing pathways to heal, move on, and change your lens in life.

In these next steps, it's essential to move slowly and take breaks, especially if you notice a lot of big emotions coming up. Remember, I say this a lot because sometimes we need continual permission to ask for help. It's also smart to have a trusted friend or professional helper nearby as you move through this process in case you need a supportive presence.

It is important to understand that this process is about reviewing your past, not reliving it. Think of the exercise like watching images of your life on a TV screen. You do not have to actually be in the events again. Detach as much as you like while you're in the review process, and stop when you feel uncomfortable or like you've reached an emotional limit.

CHANGING PARADIGMS IN ACTION

Meet Sasha, a thirty-eight-year-old woman who came to hypnotherapy seeking help for chronic self-doubt and a deep-seated fear of failure. Despite being highly competent and successful in her career as a graphic designer, Sasha felt stuck by the thought of making mistakes. She constantly overworked herself to the point of exhaustion, trying to meet her own impossibly high standards. This perfectionism was starting to take a toll on her mental and physical health.

Sasha's fear of failure and need for perfectionism stemmed from her childhood. Growing up, she had an emotionally distant father who showed approval only when she excelled academically. Her mother, a meticulous and critical woman, often pointed out Sasha's mistakes, reinforcing the belief that she was never good enough. As a result, Sasha developed the belief that her worth was tied to her achievements and that any mistake would result in rejection or disappointment.

The turning point came when Sasha was given a major project at work. Despite her team's praise and confidence in her abilities, Sasha was gripped by anxiety. She stayed up late every night, obsessively checking and rechecking her work. One evening, exhausted and overwhelmed, she broke down in tears. She realized she couldn't continue living under such immense pressure and decided to seek help.

In her hypnotherapy session, Sasha shared her feelings of inadequacy and fear of failure. Through guided visualization, she connected with her younger self—a little girl who felt loved only when she achieved something impressive. This inner child still believed that she had to be perfect to be worthy of love.

During the sessions, Sasha learned to communicate with this younger version of herself. She reassured Little Sasha that she was loved and valued just as she was, without needing to prove herself through achievements. They explored the origins of her perfectionism, understanding that it was a protective mechanism developed to cope with her parents' critical and conditional love.

As Sasha continued her hypnotherapy, she began to challenge her old beliefs. She practiced affirmations, reminding herself that she was worthy and capable regardless of her accomplishments. Gradually, she started to delegate tasks at work and set more realistic expectations for herself. She even took up painting as a hobby, allowing herself to create without the pressure of perfection.

Over time, Sasha noticed significant changes in her life. Her anxiety levels decreased, and she felt more relaxed and confident. She became more compassionate toward herself, understanding that mistakes were part of growth and not a reflection of her worth. Sasha's relationship with her parents also improved as she set boundaries and communicated her feelings more openly.

Sasha's journey illustrates how deeply ingrained beliefs from childhood can shape our perceptions and behaviors. By addressing these paradigms through hypnotherapy, she was able to shift her mindset, leading to a more balanced and fulfilling life. Her story is a testament to the power of inner work and the possibility of change, no matter how entrenched our beliefs may seem.

YOUR TURN: UNDERSTANDING YOUR PARADIGMS AND BELIEFS

Start with a few calming, centering breaths or a grounding exercise to begin to settle. Connect with your True Self before you begin this exercise so that you come from a curious, compassionate, and accepting place. Grab a journal, and try reflecting on and answering the following questions:

1. **Look at who you were in your family of origin:** What role did you play in your family? The Hero, The Jester, The Perfect One, The Scapegoat, The Screwup, The Caretaker, or something else? Look at why that role was necessary for you based on the other members of your family and the situations you experienced.

2. **Identify limiting beliefs:** What are some of the limiting beliefs you hold about yourself and your abilities? How do these beliefs impact your daily life and decisions?

3. **Trace the origins:** Can you identify specific childhood experiences or messages that contributed to these limiting beliefs and the labels you have adopted? How did these experiences shape your current perspective?

4. **Understand the emotional impact:** How do these limiting beliefs make you feel? What emotions arise when you think about them?

1. **Challenge these beliefs:** What evidence do you have that contradicts these limiting beliefs? How can you use this evidence to challenge and change your perspective?

2. **Refer back to the stages of development in Chapter 5.** Were there any big or memorable events from each of these stages of life, and how they have impacted you?

3. **Based on these events from your past**: What messages do you think you've carried with you into the present day? How do those messages affect you now? What are the beliefs you formed about yourself based on these experiences?

Reminder: Remember when I mentioned being triggered? That could come up for you as you journal. Be watchful for emotions and responses that feel bigger than what seems appropriate in the present moment. You are *not* back in that memory today. Remember that you are safe at this moment right now.

When you begin to reach back into your past, you might notice a trigger in your body. Notice how triggers show up for you so that you can reassure yourself that you're safe in the present moment—that what happened then is not happening right now, and that who you were then is not who you are now.

YOUR TURN: CONNECTING YOUR PAST TO THE PRESENT

For an additional exercise to get to know yourself, your paradigms, and your beliefs, let's explore your biography and your biology, looking at both *your* experiences and the beliefs you've inherited from previous generations.

Before you get started, choose one personal challenge or block that you wish to explore (like "Why do I feel that everything must be 'perfect' before I can relax?" or "Why do I often say yes when I really mean no?"). Some other examples of presenting issues include anxiety, people-pleasing tendencies, anger or rage, worry, a lack of confidence, or comparing yourself relentlessly to others and always coming up short.

Like you did in the last exercise, get into a safe and relaxed state and connect with your True Self–energy to support this experience. Know that your mind is there to support your highest good and won't bring to your awareness anything you aren't ready to explore. With curiosity and compassion, seek to get to know the presenting issue.

You can ask yourself: How do I sense this part of me? Does the issue bring up a feeling or an image? Is it a thought or word? Let it be whatever it is, and do your best to let go of judgment. Do your best to explore with curiosity and not judgment as you ask the presenting issue these questions: What is your role for me?" "How are you serving me?" "How do you intend to help me? Let the answers arise to the surface of your awareness without trying.

Remember that you are seeking an understanding of why this experience is part of your present life. Explore how you feel when you experience this issue. When you become deep in the weeds of your issue, do you feel lonely or unloved? Or perhaps you want approval or feel unsafe?

Next, ask what this part of you believes would happen to you or in your life if it stopped doing its job. Sit with the information that comes. Relax and soften where you can. Let go of thinking and "trying," and allow the experience to evolve organically.

When you feel complete, thank yourself, thank your body, thank your mind, and thank all the information you have received. Come back to full awareness gradually and take time to reflect and journal.

Remember, you can come back to these exercises as often as you like, and take as much time as you need to complete them. Sometimes your body will have a delayed response to the exercises I've given. You might read through a passage, try an exercise, and then days later have a "light bulb" insight or memory that tells you a little more about *why you are the way you are*—and what action you might take to encourage different behaviors and mindsets. Such is the way with any self-discovery or transformational journey.

Repeating these activities several times sends a message to your subconscious that you are ready to see and know things about yourself that may have lurked in the shadows until now. It's crucial to be gentle and accepting as new information surfaces for you.

When you stay gentle with the process, it's easier for transformation to find you and stick with you. And, as is often said in recovery circles, you may intuitively know how to handle situations that used to baffle you.

GO DEEPER AFFIRMATIONS

- I am worthy of love, success, and happiness just as I am.
- I have the power to change my beliefs and create a fulfilling life.
- I trust in my abilities and believe in my potential.

By engaging deeply with these exercises, go deeper reflection questions, and affirmations, you can uncover and begin to shift the paradigms and beliefs that have been holding you back. This inner work is essential for personal growth and transformation, allowing you to create a life that is more aligned with your True Self and your deepest desires.

Chapter 9

Forgiveness and Re-Parenting Your Inner Child

Once you've learned how your past influences your present and to connect with your inner child, you can have the power to give yourself what you did not receive back then. And how wonderful is it that despite the deficiencies in our childhood, we have the power to re-parent ourselves and supply what's missing?

It's also crucial to remember that your inner child work is not just another to-do list. You cannot treat this process like a trip to the grocery store, tick off all the food and cleaning products on your list, and then go home with neatly bagged items downloaded into your psyche. It doesn't work that way.

Before you can go get those milestones for yourself, here's an essential step you must complete first: forgiveness.

If you don't do your forgiveness work, you'll get ambushed later by resentment, guilt, shame, criticism, and judgment. All these negative emotions can keep you stuck with unhealthy habits, horrible coping skills, and big black emotional clouds that won't lift. Dissipate those clouds now so that you can clearly see your way forward.

So how do you do that? Forgiveness means letting go of any judgments, beliefs, and misunderstandings you formed from the hurts or wounds you received. When we don't let go of those negative thoughts, the pain keeps us suffering—sometimes for decades!

And you know what? You'd be perfectly justified to hold on to your blame. After all, those people, events, or circumstances really hurt you. Sometimes we resist forgiving—even ourselves—because we think there is justification to hold on to judgment.

Seriously, blame can feel like accountability! If you let go of it, does that make what happened to you okay? Does that mean that the injustice goes unnoticed? Unpunished? How do you balance the scales if you forgive?

The forgiveness we'll discuss here is first and foremost self-forgiveness. When you discover you have wounding from your childhood, it is paramount to forgive yourself for buying into negative beliefs for such a long time.

But forgiveness can be external too. It's grieving and mourning the loss of the parent you wish you had, and learning to see your caregiver as human. If this is hard, remember: they still hurt you. Forgiving your caregivers doesn't excuse their mistakes or release them from accountability. What happened to you—no matter whose "fault" it was—was not okay and never will be.

External forgiveness can also mean forgiving the systems, events, or circumstances in which you were hurt. It's recognizing what was *not* in your control, and forgiving the situation for letting you down, even though what happened to you was not okay.

When you forgive yourself and begin to see the influential adults in your early life as human beings with their own traumas, glitches, and gaps, you stop them from continuing to hurt you now, today. That way, you can move ahead with healing and filling your own gaps with the gifts you were meant to receive. When a situation in your present reminds you of a past wound, this forgiveness allows you to stop reopening that wound and reacting as if you are stuck in a younger version of yourself.

It is said that blame and resentment are like drinking poison yourself and hoping someone else will die. When you forgive yourself and the people, places, or things that hurt you, you simply stop drinking the poison so that you can finally heal. It's tempting to wait for the apology you've long sought, a reparation of some sort, or even simply an external acknowledgment that you got the short end of a developmental stick. And you're right: you deserve those things. But you don't always have control over when or whether you get them. What you do control is your own ability to move forward, and forgiveness is the first step for that.

But how do we go about forgiving ourselves and our transgressors? Like anything else worth doing well, forgiveness is a practice.

First, you must become aware of the moments when you get mired in shame, guilt, or resentment. The experience people often refer to as "being triggered" is an opportunity for that awareness.

Moments of being triggered are moments when your reaction doesn't appear to match the actual thing you're reacting to. For example, let's say some constructive feedback at work over a silly mistake sends you reeling from fear. Suddenly, you're right back to that third-grade poetry reading where you were embarrassed about your clothes and you forgot the second half of your assigned poem.

Your guts churn, your heartbeat speeds up, and you can't seem to pull it together in front of your boss. You can beat yourself up about "overreacting" to kindly meant feedback—or you can recognize that that feedback triggered a psychosocial gap.

Even though the disturbing or traumatic event is long past, you still react to triggers as if you're right there in the thick of it. This response is an invitation to explore more deeply why you're stuck so you can begin responding to your life as you are today.

Forgiveness in Action

Here is an example of how self-blame and shame can feel relentless for someone who needs to embrace self-forgiveness:

I have a client who came to me initially because she felt insecure and anxious at her job. Sally described this anxiety uptick when she had to give a presentation to a roomful of executives as part of her new promotion.

As we dove into her childhood during our initial conversation and intake, Sally shared that both of her parents were alcoholics who owned and lived at a bar. When she was six months old, her parents arranged to have her live with her babysitter permanently. As she got older, Sally would go to the bar after school to spend time with her parents and do her homework, and then would go back to her babysitter's house when the bar opened.

From an outsider's perspective, I could see how this would have had a huge effect on her confidence, self-worth, and overall belief in herself. You may also be able to imagine her feeling lonely, abandoned, pushed aside, and even super devalued because of her experience.

Sally assured me that she had done the forgiveness work. She understood that her parents had their own trauma and shortcomings, she didn't hold any grudges toward them, and she had made peace with her childhood.

That all may be true for Sally on the conscious level. However, in her hypnotherapy session, while totally relaxed, secure, and supported, she finally felt safe enough to reveal that she always felt different, not good enough, and unwanted. Sally recognized that at a very young age she thought she was the cause of her parents' arguments and therefore their drinking.

Let that sink in for a minute. That's a lot for anyone to hold deep in their body for so many years. Those beliefs have a way of saturating our very cells and coming out sideways in all sorts of sneaky behaviors and feelings.

It was no wonder her inner critic was so loud and present in her mind! Here's what that wounded voice kept whispering in Sally's ear each week:

- "If I fail, if I screw up, I will be fired." (i.e., I will be abandoned)
- "I really need to be perfect and be in control of the situation so they like me." (i.e., People will leave me if I'm not perfect.)
- "I need to fit in to be accepted, and that means not making any mistakes, not upsetting anyone." (i.e., I must keep everyone happy to be loved and valued.)

We did the big work of self-forgiveness during our time together, and Sally finally let go of the beliefs that she'd adopted during that time in her life that kept holding her back in the present day.

Then, just as important, the second step was to realize the present truth, that her inner critic was frozen in time, and had *not* grown up beyond the time it began protecting her. To protect Sally, this inner critic kept saying the same words, even though the words no longer worked to keep Sally safe and protected.

To finally release these outmoded messages, I had her complete the following two statements:

- I forgive myself for believing . . .
- The truth is . . .

In her mind, Sally imagined speaking to her inner child who first adopted the fears about abandonment and created a protector art of the inner critic. She forgave herself for developing and believing the messages her inner critic used to keep her safe. As her adult self today, she could now meet her inner child's needs that weren't met at that time. She became the parent she wished she had had. And she reminds herself of the truth often now.

For her, this went something like:

- *I forgive myself for believing I am not good enough and not lovable. I forgive myself for believing that I am unwanted and different or separate.*
- *The truth is that I am good enough, which is why I got the promotion in the first place. The truth is that I am lovable and I have a wonderful marriage to prove it. The truth is that I am wanted.*

Although we cannot go back in time and change the actual events we have experienced, we can *change our relationship with them*. And that crucial step is what this self-forgiveness practice enables you to do.

In fact, Sally's deep wounding and forgiveness, together, formed a crucible for her. This kind of crucible in your own story has the power to call you to the mat of growth, continual development, and enrichment for your whole life.

> ## YOUR TURN: FORGIVENESS
>
> Even though no one would wish tragedy or loss on themselves or someone else, imagine what a lifetime would be like with zero struggle and no challenges. Boring? Vanilla? A picture-perfect (but perhaps inauthentic, bland, and weird) existence? Though we'd all love to pick our battles, that's just not how life works. We get lemons where we least expect them. Then we get to choose whether those lemons sour our very existence or we allow forgiveness in to sweeten the whole glass of lemonade.
>
> As you move ahead on the forgiveness road, know that it, too, is an imperfect path. You'll have moments of release and deeply profound space in your head and heart one day, and the next you'll find yourself eyeballs-deep in resentment and recrimination again.
>
> Keep going. Keep repeating the healing words of forgiveness. Keep checking in with your inner child. Be the parent you wished you had had. Meet your inner child's needs when your triggers come up.
>
> Finish off those statements I wrote above ("I forgive myself for believing . . ." and "The truth is . . .") in your own healing, nourishing way—even if it feels silly and staged at first. Enlist the help of trusted others as you work to evolve your thinking and your feelings. It's even okay to repeat out loud or in your head the wrongs visited upon you. But as you say those flogging words about yourself or someone else, *follow them* with a phrase of release.

Here are some more examples in case you need to grease the forgiveness wheels a bit more (especially toward yourself):

- "Wow, I was so young and impressionable—it's no wonder I felt like the world was on my shoulders when my parents pushed me to attend all my dance classes even though I felt sick and exhausted."
- "It's okay to feel angry about what happened—but I don't have to be angry at myself."
- "Yikes! My parents really let me down and did not protect me very well. I wouldn't expect a fifteen-year-old to make good decisions about dangerous people."
- "My parents are good people who made a big mistake. I know they didn't intend to hurt me or leave me alone in a compromising situation. They really dropped the ball. I deserved to be protected then, and I just wasn't. I can protect myself and my children differently today."
- "Today I can see where I might have made the same misguided decisions, given the way each of my parents grew up. I would handle this situation a lot differently today if the tables were turned."
- "The truth is that it's not okay what happened to me."
- "The truth is that today I can get the nourishment and support I need to help me heal."
- "My caregivers made decisions based on the tools and experience they had at the time. It was not enough to protect me."
- "It's not my responsibility to change my caregivers or get them to apologize. I can assure Little Me that I'm

here for her today and that we'll heal and grow stronger together."

- "I hope that Grandma Rose can find healing and peace from the wounds that made her raise or care for me the way that she did."

Repetition is an important component on the road to shifted mindsets, self-forgiveness, and expansive feelings of peace. Your mind loves you and is always moving you toward what is familiar. Repetition makes the unfamiliar become familiar, so the more you repeat your mantras of forgiveness, the more you can finally and graciously give yourself the psychosocial gifts you deserved all along.

GO DEEPER REFLECTION QUESTIONS

- How has holding on to resentment, guilt, or shame affected your life? Consider the physical, emotional, and relational impacts.

- What would your life look like if you could fully forgive yourself and others? How might your behavior, feelings, and relationships change?

- How can you show compassion and understanding to your inner child and your present self during the process of forgiveness?

GO DEEPER AFFIRMATIONS

- I release the past and embrace forgiveness to heal my present and future.
- I forgive myself for any judgments or negative beliefs I have held about myself.
- Forgiveness empowers me to move forward with love, peace, and strength.

These reflection questions and affirmations are designed to help you delve deeper into the process of forgiveness, allowing you to release past hurts and create a more compassionate and empowered future. By engaging with these exercises regularly, you can foster a sense of peace and healing, both for your inner child and your present self.

To help strengthen your intuition "muscles," let's explore more about the life you want.

Chapter 10

Preparing for Change

Procrastination. Freezing under pressure. Never being able to speak up for what you want and need. Perfectionism. The inability to ask for help. Doing what everyone else thinks you should do without understanding what *you* want in this life.

These are all behaviors that my clients seek help to change. These clients can often see clearly that they do these things in their waking lives, but cannot understand why. And sometimes, a client comes to me because something's "off" in their life—they're not getting what they want or need—but they have no idea what the "off" thing is.

Before I can help someone behave differently (and therefore achieve different results and outcomes), I first have to help them see what's going on now, and why it's happening. Then we can do the work of unwinding the thoughts and beliefs behind the coping behavior and help them build new and supportive beliefs so they can change their actions.

Here's why this awareness step is crucial to progress. (Hint: it all goes back to the Rules of the Mind.)

We *only* do things that serve us. Therefore, the issue, habitual behavior, or quality you are experiencing that you don't want to experience anymore has served a purpose (and has actually kept you safe and secure—-if uncomfortable and unhappy—for as long as you've unconsciously used it).

It's usually true that we seek change when we recognize that our coping behaviors no longer deliver the safety and security for which we originally created them. But before lasting change can happen, you must understand how that behavior "helped" you for so long so you can find another way to meet your needs.

This is an emotional—not logical—purpose or payoff. The "why" behind your current (and undesired) behavior or quality doesn't often make logical sense when you look at it. And the rules of the mind make the undesired behavior tough to budge.

As you're uncovering and understanding the issues that keep you stuck, think about the protective strategies you possess: perfectionism, fierce inner criticism, the "controlling manager" part of you, incessant worrying, or something else that takes up a lot of your emotional time and energy. How does that behavior or thought pattern protect you? How has it kept you safe up until now? What does it shield you from?

For example, procrastination may allow you to protect yourself from failure. After all, if you never start something, you can't fail at it. According to the Principles of the Mind, if you have labeled "failure" as painful in your mind, your subconscious will do whatever it can to keep you away from the pain of failure. (Remember, your brain will always move you toward pleasure and away from pain in the ways that you define them.)

Or as another example, if *you* are your fiercest, most harshest critic, that can be a way of protecting yourself from others. No one else can cut you down more than you do to yourself. It's better to hear that criticism from yourself than from someone else, so you always beat everyone else to the punch.

There must be an understanding of what a protective strategy is protecting you *from*, as well as how and why it first emerged. Perhaps when you were little, your caregiver criticized you relentlessly. It felt awful, but you didn't have the tools or maturity to process your emotions at the time. It became easier and safer to provide the criticism internally as you grew up. You became a Perfectionist—so you had more control over the ensuing shame or sadness or anger that was too overwhelming to feel if you didn't make your caregiver happy and gain their approval.

My clients often report that their strident inner critic speaks with a voice they heard often in childhood. That voice *can* and *does* change—once it's fully understood, and once you find a healthier way to meet that same need.

In the previous example, a change in belief might look something like this, going from "I'm a total screwup—I can't make a mistake or no one will love me or stick around" to "I can love myself even when I'm not perfect. It's okay for me to be human, and I've seen over and over that my friends and loved ones will hang in there with me when I'm not perfect. I *deserve* love and belonging simply because I exist."

After you practice the new belief for a surprisingly short time, your mind will have a new paradigm for what is pain and what is pleasure. Pleasure might now be the relaxation and release of doing something imperfectly and nothing bad happening. Your brain can move you more confidently toward *more* of that feeling—and away from the exhaustion (pain) of hypervigilance against "mistakes."

Changing Your Beliefs in Action

Meet Emma, a thirty-nine-year-old marketing executive who sought out hypnotherapy after experiencing severe burnout, escalating anxiety, and recent panic attacks. Despite her successful career and outwardly perfect life, Emma was trapped in a relentless cycle of perfectionism and workaholism. She found herself constantly striving for an unattainable standard, pushing herself to the brink of exhaustion.

Emma's journey began with her desperate need for change. Her perfectionism drove her to work late nights and weekends, leaving little time for self-care or relaxation. The mounting pressure led to frequent anxiety attacks, and her once manageable stress levels spiraled into overwhelming panic attacks. Emma felt trapped, unable to break free from the relentless demands she placed on herself.

As we delved into Emma's past during our initial sessions, a clearer picture began to emerge. Emma grew up in a household where achievement and success were highly valued. Her parents, both high achievers themselves, placed immense pressure on her to excel in everything she did. Praise and affection were conditional, given only when she brought home perfect grades or excelled in extracurricular activities. This created a deep-seated belief in Emma that she was worthy of love and acceptance only if she was perfect.

In our sessions, we worked on recognizing and understanding these deeply ingrained beliefs. Emma's perfectionism was a safety strategy she developed to feel worthy and loved. However, it was now causing her significant distress and impacting her mental and physical health. Emma needed to learn to offer herself the love and acceptance she craved, regardless of her achievements.

Emma began to identify and challenge the limiting beliefs she held about her worth being tied to her achievements. She started to see how these beliefs were formed in her childhood and how they continued to influence her behavior.

We focused on cultivating self-compassion. Emma practiced self-soothing techniques and learned to be kinder to herself. She began to understand that she deserved love and acceptance simply for being herself, not for what she accomplished.

Incorporating mindfulness practices and relaxation techniques helped Emma manage her anxiety. She learned to take breaks, set boundaries, and prioritize her well-being over her work.

Emma worked on forgiving herself for the unrealistic expectations she had set. She also began to forgive her parents for the pressure they placed on her, recognizing that they were doing their best with the tools they had.

Emma's breakthrough came during a particularly intense hypnotherapy session. She visualized her younger self, a little girl desperately seeking her parents' approval. Emma embraced this inner child, reassuring her that she was loved and worthy, regardless of her achievements. This visualization allowed Emma to start healing the wounds from her past and reframing her beliefs about herself.

Over time, Emma noticed significant changes in her life. Her anxiety levels decreased, and she experienced fewer panic attacks. She started to set realistic goals and priorities, focusing on balance and self-care. Emma learned to delegate tasks at work and say no without guilt. She even rekindled her love for painting, a hobby she had abandoned in her pursuit of perfection.

Emma's journey is a testament to the power of hypnotherapy and inner work. By addressing the root causes of her perfectionism and workaholism, she was able to transform her relationship with herself and create a more balanced, fulfilling life. Today, Emma continues to nurture her well-being, knowing that her worth is intrinsic and not dependent on her achievements.

Emma's story illustrates how deeply ingrained beliefs from childhood can shape our adult lives and behaviors. Through hypnotherapy and compassionate self-reflection, it's possible to heal these wounds, shift our paradigms, and move toward a healthier, more joyful existence.

YOUR TURN: CHANGE YOUR BELIEFS

Back in Chapter 8, you connected with your inner child and learned how your past influences your present. Now we need to concisely announce what limiting beliefs you picked up and held from your childhood.

This exercise will help you identify and outline your limiting beliefs, understand their origins, and prepare for the transformative change you desire. Find a quiet, comfortable place where you can reflect without interruptions. Take a few deep breaths to center yourself and enter a state of calm focus.

1. Set the Scene: Close your eyes and take three deep, cleansing breaths. Inhale through your nose and exhale through your mouth, letting go of any tension with each exhale. Allow yourself to feel grounded and present in the moment.

2. Connect with Your True Self: Imagine a bright light at your heart center, representing your True Self—wise,

compassionate, and loving. Let this light expand, filling your entire body with warmth and love.

3. Identify Limiting Beliefs: Think about an area in your life where you feel stuck or dissatisfied. Focus on any negative thoughts or beliefs you have about yourself in this area. These could be thoughts like "I'm not good enough," "I don't deserve success," or "I'll always fail."

4. Trace the Origin: Once you've identified a limiting belief, ask yourself, "When did I first start believing this?" Allow memories from your past to surface. You might recall specific events, conversations, or general feelings from your childhood or adolescence that contributed to this belief.

5. Visualize Your Younger Self: Picture yourself at the age when this belief first formed. What were you feeling at that time? What was happening in your life? How did the people around you influence your belief?

6. Dialogue with Your Younger Self: Imagine having a conversation with this younger version of you. Ask them how they felt and why they formed this belief. Offer them compassion and understanding. Let them know that it's okay to feel the way they did.

7. Let Go of the Old Belief and Create a New Belief: Gently challenge the limiting belief and replace it with a more empowering one. For example, change "I'm not good enough" to "I am worthy and capable." Visualize your younger self accepting this new belief and feeling empowered by it.

8. Integrate the New Belief: Take a few moments to let this new belief sink in. Imagine it spreading throughout

> your body, filling you with confidence and strength. Picture yourself living with this new belief and how it positively impacts your life.

GO DEEPER REFLECTION QUESTIONS

- What are the specific limiting beliefs that you hold about yourself? How do they manifest in your thoughts, behaviors, and feelings?

- How do these limiting beliefs make you feel? What emotions arise when you think about them?

- What new, empowering beliefs would you like to adopt? How would your life change if you fully embraced these new beliefs?

GO DEEPER AFFIRMATIONS

- I deeply and completely love and accept myself.

- I see my past experiences with clarity and understand how they have shaped my beliefs.

- I embrace growth and change as a natural part of my journey.

By engaging with this exercise, reflection questions, and affirmations regularly, you can begin to uncover and shift the limiting beliefs that have been holding you back. This process will help you create a more positive, empowering mindset, paving the way for meaningful and lasting change in your life.

Chapter 11

Letting Go of Old Patterns, Emotions, and Behaviors

Even when you know a behavior, emotion, or belief has outlived its usefulness for you, how do you begin to let it go when it's so ingrained into your psyche? Into your everyday actions? Safety strategies settle into habit so subtly, sometimes, that it's hard to recognize when they're getting in your way.

Though the answer is simple, it's not always easy. You let go one observation, one pivot, one new action at a time—until the safety strategy is just another part of your past rather than your current behavior.

Believe it or not, it *is* possible to shrink your trigger buttons or eliminate them altogether, so that *all* the parts of you can feel safe most of the time. You no longer need to rely on your Protector Parts while you exile other tender parts you're ashamed of.

All the previous work of the last chapters has focused on:

- Recognizing the beliefs and behaviors that hold you back (usually housed in your Protector Parts).

- Knowing where and how those beliefs and behaviors began (to keep you safe and help you feel loved and accepted).

- Honoring the usefulness of those beliefs and behaviors for large chunks of your life (you're not broken, you're human, and this is a journey of evolution and healing, not shame or regret).

This work of discovery is crucial to the process of letting go. If you don't know what to release and how to care for all of your parts in the process, after all, you'll never feel safe trying to force change. And the change you want will not last, even if you succeed in temporarily altering your course.

It's also natural to intentionally release an emotion or belief, only to claw it back into your existence later on when you feel triggered or unsafe. Letting go is a process and a practice, just like meditation, mindfulness, or exercise. The more you do it, the easier and more automatic it gets, sort of like brushing your teeth.

When you can recognize that these beliefs you've held about yourself ("I'm unlovable," "I'm not enough," "The only way I receive love and validation is through achievement," etc.) are driving your unwanted behaviors, you can see they are no longer true.

You have the power to release the beliefs that are no longer serving you. When you developed those punishing inner beliefs, you didn't have the resources you have now. With self-compassion, offer yourself forgiveness for believing these things in the first place. Instead, recognize what is actually true now.

By the way, what *is* true about you, now that you've read about how early beliefs take hold?

It's true that:

- You're human—prone to mistakes, messes, challenges, triumphs, and everything in between. And it is all good.
- You deserve to feel loved and accepted just because you exist.
- Perfection is not required in order to gain belonging, nurturing, and satisfaction in your life.
- Rest and recovery are paramount to your life's fulfillment—guilt-free.
- Joy is your birthright.

Believing the above list is another matter entirely. Believing these *new* inner messages is a practice, just like letting go of the old ones. It can be deeply helpful to have an action—a ceremony, of sorts—to assist in the practice of letting go of the old and welcoming in the new.

Some of my clients really enjoy creating and practicing ceremonies to mark life milestones and help in their "letting go" process. Other clients prefer to keep it simple and quick. Regardless of your ceremonial preference, it *is* crucial to give yourself some kind of practice to separate yourself from your old beliefs, no matter how often they crop up.

Your ceremony can be solely in your mind as a "letting go" visualization (like seeing your old beliefs floating swiftly down a river, or mentally throwing them in a trash can, or tying them to a brick and dropping them off a tall building.) Or it can be something you act out safely in real life.

LETTING GO IN ACTION

Here's how my client Camila approached the task of letting go. Camila came to me with a successful career, happy marriage, and a severe autoimmune condition that caused her to lose patches of her hair and suffer burning sensations on her skin and scalp. She visited me after the second significant flare-up on this condition, each one following a stressful time in her career where she got devastatingly burned out.

Camila had put a lot of pressure on herself her whole life. In high school, she became an athlete, took on a second language, and sang in the choir. Camila and her sister were ruthlessly competitive in all areas, and her home life was chaotic, plus she never knew when her mother would explode in an angry tirade and clamp down with stifling strictness.

In our session together, Camila realized that she'd never felt worthy of her mom's love because her mom had never offered it to her. She could only feel worthy of acceptance when she won the big game, sang like a rock star, or aced the exam. Only achievement and performance would give her validation, attention, and the feeling she was good enough.

With this realization, Camila connected the dots of her early development with her current need to have everything look perfect—her marriage, career, and success. She could see how she was working so hard to be "enough," despite not really believing it was possible for her.

No matter what new success she claimed or shiny thing she owned, she still believed she had to work to utter exhaustion to have worth, to be loved, and to belong. And her body simply wasn't having it any longer, hence the skin flares, hair loss, and body pain.

Remember that your mind will always lead you toward validating your inner beliefs in your outer world; it's your Protector Parts resorting to the coping skills they've always employed to keep you "safe," even when it's uncomfortable, painful, or harmful to you.

With a gentle "aha!" Camila recognized that these beliefs were not true. She was ready to let them go and call in new ones.

After our session, we reinforced her discoveries with a personalized hypnosis recording. As she listened to it several times in the coming weeks, Camila got consistent reminders that she didn't have to perform to get the love and belonging she needed. She was able to let go of the belief that she was only worthy if she was achieving. She replaced those beliefs with ones like:

- "I am worthy of love and care."
- "I can rest and recover and still enjoy belonging."
- "Love is mine because I exist."

Camila reported that the autoimmune symptoms greatly reduced in the weeks following our session. She also took inspired action to lessen her workload and dial back on career pressure—guilt-free.

YOUR TURN: LETTING GO RITUALS

Here are two ceremonies you can try on your own as a way to release old, limiting beliefs and call in new, expansive ones.

Burning of Grievances:

- Once you've uncovered your loudest limiting beliefs from Chapter 10, write them down, each on their own piece of paper. Intentionally crumple each of these papers.

- Find a large fire-safe container and head outside to a calm place where you can enjoy peaceful solitude. You might also choose to bring a couple of witnesses with you, like close friends or family.

- Take one of your crumpled belief-papers, place it in the container, and light it on fire.

- Watch each paper turn to ash, one at a time.

- Recognize they are permanently gone from your life. You can never get them back, even if you wanted to.

If Fire Isn't Your Thing:

- Use a bit of sugar to represent each belief. Spoonful by spoonful, dissolve the sugar into a cup of water. Once it's dissolved, pour the water down the drain and see it washing away from your life and experience, permanently.

- Or imagine your next shower is a cleansing ritual, washing away any old, outdated, limiting beliefs.

Important note for all of these rituals: Be sure to recognize the permanent state of the letting go. You cannot get back the papers from the ashes or the water from down the drain. Similarly, you cannot get back the old beliefs. They can no longer negatively impact you once they are permanently gone from your subconscious mind and your body.

GO DEEPER REFLECTION QUESTIONS

- What emotions are you holding on to from past experiences? How do these emotions affect your current state of mind and behavior?

- How can you reinterpret past events to find a sense of peace and acceptance? What positive lessons or strengths have you gained from these experiences?

GO DEEPER AFFIRMATIONS

- I release the weight of my past and embrace the freedom of the present.

- I allow myself to heal from old wounds and open my heart to new possibilities.

- I accept my past and its lessons, knowing they have shaped me into who I am today.

Whew! We're nearly complete with our therapeutic journey together . . . for now. Your recovery and healing are an ongoing process. It's paramount to normalize the many layers of growth and evolution we all experience in one human life.

The good news is that as you build these new beliefs inside you, it's much easier and faster to course-correct when you hit inevitable triggers over time. The acute discomfort and stuckness you go through at the very beginning of your transformation become less fraught and more manageable.

Eventually the Protector Parts that resorted to outmoded coping skills at the slightest hint of danger will become your allies—helping you recognize the work you've done, the strides you've made, and your innate ability to comfort, support, and regulate yourself in ways that keep feeding your progress, without sending you into the red zone of fight-flight-freeze.

Chapter 12

New Roles for Your Old Parts

So what happens to your Protector Parts after you move through a deep healing process? Do they simply wander off in your mind, retiring to greener pastures? Do you still need them? Is it possible for an out-of-work Protector Part to learn new job skills and go through a complete "career change" after vigilantly looking after you for so long?

The short answer is yes. Just like a human can very happily change careers and still be relevant and fulfilled and feel super useful, so can your Protector Parts. They will always be there for you as a crucial part of your psyche, just in a job for which they are better suited, a job that wasn't developed out of necessity. You still get to keep all the positive qualities and patterns that your Protector Part may have gifted you along the way. The new role integrates everything you love about your Protectors and none of the negative outcomes of their well-intentioned hypervigilance

Here's how to offer your Protector Parts a smooth transition into . . . something else.

You've done a lot of work over the previous chapters:

- Understanding the role of each pattern

- Working with the inner child, letting go of the past beliefs
- Forgiving yourself

Now, you'll need to reconnect with the original presenting issue and see how it feels in your body.

Let's say your presenting issue is perfectionism. How does it feel to you now that the towels may not be folded as precisely as you would like, someone else has loaded the dishwasher, and the spreadsheet didn't add up as neatly as you wished?

Observe how your body feels knowing that several tasks aren't done the way you prefer. If (for now) your stomach is calm, if you can focus on another activity you enjoy, and if you can set aside your to-do list while you sink fully into a deep hug from your partner, that's amazing progress.

If you still feel the tug of your Protector Parts, like your Perfectionist pushing you into the "safety" of hyper-functioning, it's time to talk to that part again so that you don't feel so exhausted dealing with those old protective patterns. It's imperative to help your Protector Part (the Perfectionist, in this case) see that the greater Self (*you*, in other words) is now in charge of all of your parts, even the Perfectionist Part. If the Perfectionist can see and understand this internal power shift, they may see that they don't need to work so hard to protect the entire system.

When you notice harsh inner messaging and frantic action cropping up, take a quiet moment and ask your inner critic if it still feels it needs the same job as before. Ask if it's ready to support you in a different way that feels nourishing and restorative, not punishing. Remind this part that *you* (the Self—the one in charge) can take care of the system as a whole without the old protective strategies. Even a simple action like putting your hand on your heart and whispering, "We are safe, I've got this," can disarm your Protector Parts.

Sometimes that part is ready to change—your inner critic turns into your inner cheerleader with just a little encouragement and reassurance. Other times, you may need to negotiate for a shift with your Protector Part at a later time. You can move the process along by asking additional questions of your Protector Part like:

- "What do you need in order to feel like you're ready to relinquish your role?"
- "What needs to happen in my life for you to feel safe?"

Your Protector Part may answer back something like:

- "I need you to create stronger, healthier boundaries with our mom so that I don't feel so activated when she stays at the house too long and then starts criticizing the way we vacuum the carpet."
- "I need you to silence the notifications on your phone after work so I don't snap to attention when I hear your email alarm go off and I can unplug from constant achievement while valuing our downtime."
- "I need a lot of deep rest and recovery because I've worked so hard for so long to keep you safe—I'm just really tired."

Protector Reassignment in Action

I met with Elizabeth over a few sessions. She worked in a high-powered corporate position but lacked confidence. Her homelife had changed drastically with her recent divorce, and she was adjusting to single parenthood with two children.

Elizabeth's self-doubt resulted in endless inner comparison to her male counterpart, who seemed to be the boss's favorite. Because of all the imposter syndrome going on inside her, Elizabeth procrastinated on projects (what if she didn't complete them perfectly?), avoided presentations (what if she looked stupid or incompetent?), and self-sabotaged her success (if she rejected herself, it would protect her from the potential rejection of others).

Through the same process I've shared in this book, Elizabeth and I tracked the self-doubt, lack of confidence, and the silent shame she was experiencing. They all had messages for her, and it was my job to help her decode the messages and replace them with positive voices.

Elizabeth asked to get to know the self-doubt part. When was it created? What did it feel it needed to protect?

The answer that came through was that the self-doubt part protected Elizabeth's inner child. When she was a little girl, Elizabeth lived in the shadow of her high-achieving older sister. Elizabeth watched from the sidelines as her sister received all the family attention, love, and acceptance for her continuing accolades.

This self-doubt part of Elizabeth took on the role of Protector to keep her safe from rejection, embarrassment, humiliation, and failure. As a child, Elizabeth quickly learned that by staying small and quiet, she felt safer, because what if she never measured up to her bright and shining older sister? While this self-doubt part did its job incredibly well in childhood, self-doubt had long overstayed its usefulness in her life as an adult.

Elizabeth found a way to rescue her inner child from behind the self-doubt Protector Part by meeting her inner child's needs and keeping her safe. This shift happened over months filled with small actions, like:

- Listening to our recorded session each day to check in with her inner child

- Witnessing her inner child's experience from long ago (because she did not feel seen or validated when she was little)

- Doing activities now that she loved to do as a child, like coloring, being outside, and dancing

- Catching herself responding to real-life moments as her wounded inner child

- Taking a deep breath with a hand on her heart and stomach while assuring the inner child that she was safe, and that Elizabeth was taking care of her

Once Elizabeth's self-doubt part could see that Elizabeth's inner child was safe with Elizabeth, it could take on the new role of confident inner cheerleader.

Elizabeth created her own practice to build trust, security, and belonging with her inner child. She let go of the old, outdated beliefs that she was not important, that she was less than her siblings, and that she had to be quiet to be safe.

She called in new, more powerful beliefs that she was worthy and valuable, that people wanted to hear what she had to say, and that her voice deserved to be heard. Tending to her inner child every day helped her make this shift.

She forgave herself for buying into those old, worn-out beliefs in the first place, knowing that at the time, they did serve her, but now they were holding her back. She checked back with the self-doubt part, and it was finally ready to change roles.

YOUR TURN: REASSIGN PROTECTOR PARTS

Let's build on the work of the previous activities and gently de-role your Protector Part.

- Prior to this activity, be sure to review the exercises you've completed from the previous chapters, especially the ones where you got to know a part and your inner child, and the "letting go" exercises you worked through on your own. These steps remain important to have in mind when "negotiating" a new role for a part.

- Get into a comfy meditative state, like sitting in a supportive chair, or lying on a mat or blanket on the floor. Choose to close your eyes or soften your gaze based on your comfort.

- Connect with your True Self—cultivate the qualities of compassion, caring, and curiosity.

- Looking inward, check back with the part of you that you worked with previously.

- Notice the sensations, color, texture, and images that you associate with this part. Recognize if it feels or shows up differently from when you first worked with it.

- Remember, this part has witnessed the work you have done and all of the healing you have gone through as you have read this book and done the activities.

- Thank the part for showing up and sharing with you. And thank the part for helping you in the way it has.

- Ask the part, "With the healing I've been through, do you still need the old role of____?"

- If it says no, ask it what it would like to do instead.

- If it says yes, ask it what it would need from you to let go of the role in the future.

- If this need is something you can agree to, make a commitment to this part to provide it so that the part can let go of its role and try something more supportive.

- Once you come to an agreement, thank this part again. Come back to your True Self.

- Take a few breaths and gradually awaken into full awareness.

- Spend a few moments writing what you experienced in your journal. You can use the following questions to help guide you if needed:

  - Is the part ready to take on a new role?

  - What did you need to do to satisfy the commitment to this part?

  - Write down a few statements of gratitude for this part.

  - What are some of the positive qualities you gained from the part's protective strategies that you'd like to keep?

It's okay to revisit and perhaps even enjoy your journaling and your journey along the path to total acceptance of this part (and *all* your parts.) They are essential pieces of the beautiful human being that is *you*, after all.

Always remember that you are *not* broken. There is no fatal flaw here to correct. All of your parts have or had purpose in your life—to keep you safe, to keep you loved, to help you belong.

When we understand that there is a True Self we can call on to manage and shepherd all of our parts into healthy service to our lives, we are finally *free* to evolve. With the help of our True Self and all our parts, we can flourish, take up space, and *live* into our dreams for meaningful relationships, work that fuels us, and play that fills us to the brim with happiness and contentment. Welcome to your one, precious life.

Chapter 13

Getting the Life You Want

Perhaps the most poignant part of doing the work of healing is knowing precisely what kind of life you want, but recognizing that you have been missing the mark. That's where many programs come up short—you dig to understand *why you are the way you are* . . . but then don't take the strategic and supported action to get you where you want to ultimately go.

Many of my clients come to see me for stress relief, confidence, building financial abundance, changing their bodies, advancing in their careers, or improving their relationships—all worthy goals for sure. Some clients also come to me for help with their perfectionism, people-pleasing, lack of self-worth, codependency, or feeling like they are "not enough." Hypnosis can help you restructure the inner messaging that keeps you stuck in either internal battles or external quagmires, and get you moving toward your version of a "better" life through strategic action.

To achieve the results you want, it is essential to shovel into your past. Along the way, you'll discover how your inner critic shows up and what sort of voice it has. It's also paramount to recognize and accept every big or small trauma you endured, challenge you faced, or "mistake" you made along the way.

Reminder: Looking at your past is about reviewing it, not reliving it. Reviewing your past is about stopping the fight with reality. Don't spend all your energy wishing it never happened. Spend your energy on what you can do now.

But to truly transform yourself and your situation, action is required. The first step is knowing precisely where you want to go. It's usually not enough to simply say, "I wish I could relax and cut myself a break!" or "I should just stop comparing myself to everyone else." (If only it were that easy, right?) Real change takes specificity and vision. The more detail you can add to your vision of a "better" life, the more likely you'll be to act to make that picture real.

Here's why creating a clear vision is essential for making progress:

- It is motivating to "see" the details of your ideal life. You'll know when you're moving closer to your goal or further away.
- You'll stay focused. Humans notoriously get distracted. A vision for yourself keeps you on track and taking the necessary actions for progress.
- It's easier to make the "right" choices when you have a picture of your destination in mind. (When you know you're headed to the rocky red-brown deserts of Arizona, you'll recognize very quickly if you lose your way in the midst of a mossy green swamp in Louisiana.)

Important note: It's more important to get clear on the characteristics and feelings you want to embody than the specific outcomes of your vision. For example, when you say, "I want to be a fearless, creative, inspired person," there are many ways for that vision to come true. Avoid limiting yourself with statements like "I want to sell my artwork," which gives you only *one* possible outcome.

The Neuroscience of Manifesting Your Desired Outcomes

So, how do we turn ideas and visions into real events, accomplishments, and progress? It's simple science. Let's take a look at the physiology of bringing "better" into your life.

Recent research by Dr. Carol Dweck suggests that if you believe you can do something, you're way more likely to do it than if you don't have that belief. And belief is a huge part of the hypnotherapeutic process. So it makes sense that clearing out old, conflicting beliefs is the very first step in the process of manifestation. It's imperative to allow your mind to believe that you deserve the life you envision

Think about it. If the voice in your head tells you you'll surely fail at a particular accomplishment, it can seem a lot harder to move toward success. If you believe you'll fail, then why even try? However, if you believe you can achieve a particular outcome, you're more likely to do the work required to get you closer to your goal (or recognize and say yes to the opportunities that get you closer to your goal).

And let's not confuse this belief-equals-success phenomenon with the Law of Attraction, a popular New Age lens on getting what you want out of life. The Law of Attraction says that if you believe something deeply enough, it will simply materialize in your reality as if by magic.

The Life You Want in Action

Science suggests that our positive beliefs about an outcome link us to the motivation, action, and follow-through required to bring about the desired result. An example might look something like this:

A woman comes to see me and desperately wants to spend and enjoy more time with her family and friends, but she feels overwhelmed by and anxious about her miles-long to-do list. She cannot rest or allow herself any enjoyment until all the tasks are finished, but they are never finished. Her kids miss her and do not really know her. Her partner has given up on getting her to change. She can annoy her friends and family with her relentless doing until everything is perfect and checked off the list. If she does take time for herself, she feels she'll let someone down, and she cannot live with that.

Before she can change anything, she must envision the life she actually wants to live. It could be a picture of her laughing on the beach in the sun, playing in the waves with her children or partner.

Or perhaps enjoying a backyard BBQ that she did not plan or prepare—she's off the hook for any task and is completely unworried as she talks companionably with her friends, holds hands with her partner, and eats all the yummy food on her plate, guilt-free.

Or even sitting at her desk at work, totally enjoying feeling like she matters, that her job fulfills her and challenges her without being overwhelming—that her team has her back no matter what and they communicate, job-share, and champion each other every week.

When this woman can see the vision, it also becomes clear what healing practices, mindset shifts, and actions may be required of her to get to that vision.

So, Belief = Willingness to Do the Work Required. And the "work" is what brings about the result. Plus, when the belief is strong enough, the action required for the outcome often feels less like work and more like something completely organic, intuitive, or even joyful—even though the process of getting what you want can still be challenging or trigger nervousness or fear.

It's crucial to remember that the same process works in reverse. If you do not believe that you can have the outcome you want, you'll likely engage in actions or behaviors that ensure you won't get that outcome. Our beliefs are powerful compasses. It's crucial to set them accurately on the course we most want to follow.

We cannot discuss and create your vision without a parallel chat about your "why," as in, Why this change? Why now? Spoiler alert: If the answer is anything other than a deep desire within yourself, it's likely that the vision you set will not come to pass. If you're trying to make a change to please, caretake, or appease someone outside of you, it just won't work.

My story from the beginning is a prime example of creating a life for reasons outside of a true why. I made many decisions about my life based on what I thought I "should" be doing as I described in the beginning of the book. That did not serve me well and led to dissatisfaction.

And by the way, we all make millions of decisions to please someone else; it's often a part of a safety strategy we developed in childhood. When our safety strategies start to feel anything other than safe, though, it's time to look closely at our reasons for keeping them.

You'll sabotage yourself in your quest for transformation if you are not attached to the "why" of the change you desire. When your goals do not spring from within your deepest, grandest, highest desires for you and only you, they are doomed to remain on the shelf at best, or tear down you and the people you care about at worst.

When you connect deeply to the "why" of your desired change, it becomes the intrinsic motivation that keeps you chugging ahead and making progress even when feelings get big and overwhelming, old baggage comes to the surface, and the going gets tough.

For example, a deep "why" for getting sober might be, "My body feels horrible when I drink, I'm tired of feeling tired all the time, I want to like myself more than I do right now, and I deserve to feel good." And a "why" that might backfire could sound like, "If I stop drinking so much my partner may be less upset with me—and everyone says I should cut down."

Or how about a career context? Here's a "why" that won't work: "I have to be successful and make more money so that my father will finally be proud of me, I'll have more friends, and I can buy a bigger house. Then I'll be good enough."

Here's a "why" that could better grease the wheels of your manifestation: "I am being underpaid for my skill level, I'm ready to contribute more to my team, and I'd love some leadership experience."

Whew! Now that we have the hard stuff out of the way . . .

YOUR TURN: ENVISION THE LIFE YOU WANT

Here's an activity that can help you shape a vision of the life you'd like to have. Have some fun with this one—it's where you and your imagination get to play together. Whatever you do, try not to censor yourself or remind yourself why your vision could never happen. The point here is to play with possibilities—and believe me, anything is possible with a clear vision in mind! (I've seen just about everything from my clients, so I hope you'll trust me when I say you can have what you want.)

The Sky's the Limit (A Dream-Life Exploration)

Grab a pen. You can even write everything down right here on these pages if you like. The following are my favorite questions to ask to get your imaginative and visionary juices flowing. For the next few minutes, set aside all your inner restrictions, disbelief, or self-critical thoughts. (Don't worry, they'll be right there for you when you're done—if you still want to pick them back up.)

There's no pressure to answer every question. Instead, pick the ones that feel the most open, juicy, or creative for you and be sure to list all the details you like. I'll see you on the other side of your vision.

1. If you could have anything you wanted in life, what would it be?
2. What kind of person do you want to be?
3. What are your deepest values and how do you want to align your life with them?
4. What kind of impact do you want to make in the world?
5. What kind of legacy do you want to leave behind?
6. What is the most important thing you want to accomplish in your lifetime?
7. What are your greatest fears and how can you overcome them?
8. How do you want to be remembered by others?

9. What kind of people do you want to surround yourself with?

10. What does true happiness and fulfillment mean to you?

11. How do you want to feel on a daily basis?

12. What emotions or mental states do you want to cultivate in your life?

13. What kind of relationship do you want to have with yourself?

14. How do you want to handle stress, disappointment, and setbacks?

15. What kind of personal growth do you want to achieve?

16. How do you want to balance your work, family, and personal life?

17. What kind of spiritual or philosophical beliefs do you want to incorporate into your life?

18. How do you want to maintain a sense of balance and harmony in your life?

19. What kind of self-care practices do you want to implement to support your well-being?

20. How do you want to continue to evolve and grow as a person?

Now that you have your vision fleshed out, it's time to get moving toward that vision—one itty-bitty step at a time. Hypnotherapy can support you moving toward the vision you've just described by shifting the beliefs that drive your next actions.

Though we're coming to the end of our time together in this book, let's take one more chapter to ensure you have the support and guidance you need to make change happen in your life.

Chapter 14

So What Now? (Hint: Support, Integration, Consistency)

So what now? You've finished this book, done all the exercises, and you can expect your life to be grand and problem-free from this point forward, right?

Well, no. (Best not to sugarcoat the inevitable.) The bad news is that healing is an ongoing, many-layered process. The *good news*, however, is that healing is an ongoing, many-layered process. It gets easier to evolve the more you practice, reset old mindsets, and replace outmoded inner beliefs with helpful, uplifting ones.

Even if you are the most deliberate, disciplined person in the world when it comes to healing practices, you'll grind against the feeling of taking two steps forward and one step back. You'll get stuck again. You'll wonder if you've really done any growing at all when the going gets tough, as it certainly will for all of us beautiful humans.

And of course, new challenges and triggers can erupt at any time. Life is like that. You'll still have to navigate every day, every week, every year a little at a time, and you'll have to feel all kinds of emotions and rise above evolving circumstances.

The key is to put the yardstick behind you from time to time so that you can see just how far you've come. Even as you finish this book, you cannot unknow what you've come to know here in these pages. Your life is different—is continually changing—as a simple result of reading. A. Book. (Whoa!)

Here are some other "gremlins" you may notice pop up in the coming weeks as you put some space between you and this material:

- **Resistance:** You may feel resistance to the new ideas to which you've been exposed. Your inner critic may call this process silly, or discredit the work you've done so far.

- **Disbelief:** *"How is this hypnotherapy thing supposed to work, anyway? Isn't it just a bunch of new age hoo-ha?"* Watch for this and other similar statements from inside you. These thoughts are likely messages from a part of you that still feels defensive, hurt, or anxious. Try some of the exercises we've done together so far, and see if you can shift that part to a more relaxed and willing helper to your process.

- **Lack of follow-through:** Sure, you can read a book and feel a little better while you're buried in the pages. But the real work happens when you take the ideas and practices here and apply them to your life from time to time, to actually *change yourself* from the inside out.

I know that you want your life to continue to feel better long after you put this book down. But I hope you'll continue to revisit the material when you feel uncertain, unclear, or frustrated with your progress. The same exercises will always be here for you—ready to deliver their uplifting, restful, or transformative gifts each time you practice them.

And the best news is that after practicing the tools I've given you in this book, you're more likely to navigate new challenges in different ways that get you through the tough times more quickly and easily. What seemed excruciatingly hard to deal with in the past may in fact become easier and less stressful as it pops up again in your life.

Here's how to keep your evolution going—gently, but consistently.

- Patience, compassion, and grace are all needed in the after-healing phase. You'll slip back into old ways of thinking. Your various parts are still vulnerable to triggers. It's okay. Simply notice what's going on as soon as you can, and then try employing some of your new skills as you're able. Everyone moves at their own pace.

- Your mind loves what is familiar and comfortable. Through the healing work, you are asking your mind to change, so it is important to continue to do the work. Remind yourself that you are worthy, you are deserving, and you are enough. Your mind will respond to those messages with time and practice, and your trigger buttons *will* eventually shrink and maybe even disappear altogether.

- Continue to connect with your inner child. Frequent check-ins help ensure your inner child doesn't feel forgotten, abandoned, or unimportant to you. You can increase your feelings of value and worthiness by turning toward the inner child often.

- Seek out support if you feel you aren't able to complete the healing journey on your own, or if you need an expert to help you go into more depth. Sometimes a book is all you need. Often, a book will open a door to larger healing opportunities. Be courageous. You found this material for a reason. If you read this far and still feel like there's more work to do, it's likely because you're *ready* to undertake that work.

- When other triggers come up for you, revisit the process in this book.

Ultimately, It's Always Your Turn . . .

Remember always that you're the exact right person at the exact right time. You are whole and complete just as you are. And your evolution and healing will proceed as you become ready.

I'm with you, here for you, and cheering you on all the way, and so are all of your beautiful, functional, essential parts.

So, go forth in strength, courage, and the knowledge that you've gained here in these pages. Remember, you are your own best expert, even if you need and want guidance and support in getting to that expertise.

You now have tools for healing that you didn't before. Go within. Speak to all your beautiful parts—let them share their voices with you, instead of having to manipulate and control you with their protective behaviors. They will change when you give them a chance.

You've got this. I'm with you. Be well, and be inspired to always keep evolving.

—with ALL the love,

Sara

Continue the Work with Private Hypnotherapy

If you felt inspired by this book and want to continue the work with me in private hypnotherapy, here's how to get in touch and schedule your first session:

www.themindfulmovement.com/sara

For Further Reading

- *No Bad Parts: Healing Trauma and Restoring Wholeness with the Internal Family Systems Model* by Richard C. Schwartz PhD

- *Introduction to Internal Family Systems (Second Edition)* by Richard Schwartz PhD

- *Hakomi Mindfulness-Centered Somatic Psychotherapy: A Comprehensive Guide to Theory and Practice* by Editors Halko Weiss, Greg Johanson, and Lorena Monda

- *Altered Traits: Science Reveals How Meditation Changes Your Mind, Brain, and Body* by Daniel Goleman and Richard J. Davidson

- *You Are the Placebo: Making Your Mind Matter* by Dr. Joe Dispenza

- *Mind to Matter: The Astonishing Science of How Your Brain Creates Material Reality* by Dawson Church

www.ingramcontent.com/pod-product-compliance
Ingram Content Group UK Ltd.
Pitfield, Milton Keynes, MK11 3LW, UK
UKHW020656240225
4724UKWH00048B/387